Operative
Paediatric
Urology

Operative Paediatric Urology

EDITED BY

J. DAVID FRANK MB FRCS
Consultant Paediatric Surgeon and Urologist,
Bristol Royal Hospital for Sick Children,
Bristol, UK

J. H. JOHNSTON MB FRCS FRCSI FACS FAAP
Formerly Lecturer in Paediatric Urology,
University of Liverpool and Urological Surgeon,
Alder Hey Children's Hospital, Liverpool, UK

ILLUSTRATIONS BY
PHILIP WILSON FMAA AIMI

Churchill Livingstone

EDINBURGH LONDON MELBOURNE AND NEW YORK 1990

CHURCHILL LIVINGSTONE
Medical Division of Longman Group UK Limited

Distributed in the United States of America by
Churchill Livingstone Inc., 1560 Broadway, New
York, N.Y. 10036, and by associated companies,
branches and representatives throughout the
world.

First Edition 1990

ISBN 0 443 034788

British Library Cataloguing in Publication Data
Operative paediatric urology.
  1. Children. Urogenital system. Surgery
  I. Frank, J. David   II. Johnston, J. H. (James Herbert)
  617'.46'0088054

Library of Congress Cataloging in Publication Data
Operative paediatric urology/edited by J. David Frank, J.H.
  Johnston.—1st ed.
      p.   cm.
    ISBN 0-443-03478-8
    1. Genitourinary organs—Surgery.   2. Pediatric urology.
  I. Frank, J. David.   II. Johnston, J. Herbert (James Herbert)
    [DNLM: 1. Urogenital System—surgery.   2. Urologic Diseases—in
infancy & childhood.   WS 320 061]
  RD571.066   1990
  617.4'61—dc20
  DNLM/DLC
  for Library of Congress   89-24013
                                                                CIP

Printed and bound in Great Britain by
William Clowes Limited, Beccles and London

We are well aware that operative surgery relating to any specialty cannot be learned simply from studying a textbook, even when superbly illustrated, any more than reading *Larousse Gastronomique* can make one a chef de cuisine. Nevertheless, we believe that the present volume will be of value to those surgeons, whether of paediatric surgical or urological affiliation (or in certain circumstances of both or neither), who wish to learn the preferred modern methods of correction of genito-urinary disorders in children.

We have omitted descriptions of endoscopic techniques since in our view these do not lend themselves to useful pictorial representation. Our aim has been to discuss and portray operative methods specific to paediatric problems although not necessarily needing to be performed during childhood. Urological procedures which are technically similar at all ages, such as renovascular surgery and operations for urinary calculi, have not been included.

An exhaustive description of every means of correction of the various lesions we could have discussed would have led to the production of a multi-volumed encyclopaedia. For that reason we have asked our expert contributors to describe the methods they have found to be most successful and, therefore, to be recommended to others.

An essential contribution to the book is that of our artist, Philip Wilson. We are indebted to him not only for his most excellent drawings but also for his ready and sympathetic understanding of the difficulty surgeons can often experience in depicting their operative techniques in easily comprehensible two-dimensional terms.

The book has had a lengthy gestation, to the extent that no fewer than six representatives of Churchill Livingstone have in succession held responsibility for its production. Its ultimate delivery was carried out by Mr Simon Fathers. We are grateful to him and his colleagues for their advice, their endurance and their continued enthusiasm.

We would also like to thank Mrs Carole Sweet for all her diligence in the preparation of this manuscript.

Bristol and Formby 1990   J.D.F.
                                                                           J.H.J.

A. Bianchi MD FRCS FRCS(Ed)
Consultant Paediatric Surgeon, Royal Manchester Children's Hospital, Pendlebury, UK

Kevin A. Burbige MD
Columbia-Presbyterian Medical Center, Babies Hospital, New York, USA

S. Joseph Cohen MB BCh FRCS MRCP
Formerly Lecturer in Paediatric Surgery, University of Manchester; Consultant Paediatric Surgeon and Urologist, Booth Hall Children's Hospital, Royal Manchester Children's Hospital and Saint Mary's Hospital, Manchester, UK

John W. Duckett MD
Professor of Urology and Surgery, University of Pennsylvania School of Medicine; Director, Division of Pediatric Urology, Children's Hospital of Philadelphia, Philadelphia, USA

J. David Frank MB FRCS
Consultant Paediatic Surgeon and Urologist, Bristol Royal Hospital for Sick Children, Bristol, UK

John P. Gearhart MD FAAP FACS
Assistant Professor of Pediatric Urology, Johns Hopkins University School of Medicine; Assistant Director of Pediatric Urology, James Buchanan Brady Urological Institute, The Johns Hopkins Hospital, Baltimore, USA

Terry W. Hensle MD FACS FAAP
Associate Professor of Clinical Urology, Columbia University College of Physicians and Surgeons; Director, Pediatric Urology, Babies Hospital, Columbia-Presbyterian Medical Center, New York, USA

J. H. Johnston MB FRCS FRCSI FACS FAAP
Formerly Lecturer in Paediatric Urology, University of Liverpool; Urological Surgeon, Alder Hey Children's Hospital, Liverpool, UK

A. R. Mundy MS FRCS MRCP
Senior Lecturer in Urology, the United Hospitals Medical School and the Institute of Urology; Consultant Urological Surgeon, Guy's Hospital and the St. Peter's Hospitals, London, UK

Contributors

Alberto Pena MD
Professor of Surgery and Chief Pediatric Surgeon, Schneider Children's
Hospital, Long Island Jewish Medical Center, New York, USA

A. M. K. Rickwood BM FRCS
Paediatric Urological Surgeon, Royal Liverpool Children's Hospital,
Alder Hey, Liverpool, UK

Howard M. Snyder III MD
Associate Professor of Surgery and Urology, University of
Pennsylvania School of Medicine; Associate Director, Division of
Pediatric Urology, Children's Hospital of Philadelphia, USA

Timothy P. Stephenson MS FRCS
Consultant Urological Surgeon, Cardiff Royal Infirmary, Cardiff, UK

Robert H. Whitaker MD MChir FRCS
Consultant Paediatric Urologist, Addenbrooke's Hospital, Cambridge,
UK

Contents

Contents

Chapter 1

Pyeloplasty

J. D. Frank

Introduction

The majority of patients with a pelvi-ureteric junction (PUJ) obstruction present with symptoms. The decision as to whether or not the obstruction is severe enough to require surgical repair in such cases is not difficult to make. The advent of antenatal diagnoses of PUJ obstructions using maternal ultrasound has made this decision more difficult. These babies are asymptomatic and thriving. There is a wide spectrum in the severity of the obstruction and recently Ransley & Manzoni (1985) have shown that drainage may improve postnatally with conservative management alone. Thus, in these equivocal cases, more sophisticated techniques of investigation are required to decide whether surgery is indicated.

DIAGNOSIS AND INVESTIGATIONS

The symptoms of a PUJ obstruction are usually those of flank pain often associated with vomiting. Occasionally urinary tract infection and haematuria are presenting features. All such patients should be screened with an ultrasound examination of the kidneys. If the presence of a hydronephrosis is confirmed, the absolute diagnosis of a PUJ obstruction is made using either a dynamic renal scan (e.g. DTPA) or an intravenous urogram. If a hydronephrosis is not detected but the clinical suspicion of an intermittent obstructive uropathy remains, investigations should be repeated with a water load or during an attack of pain. If the kidney is poorly functioning it may be difficult to define the exact site of obstruction using these investigations. An antegrade pyelogram with or without pressure studies may then be required. The decision as to whether to proceed to a pyeloplasty or a nephrectomy of a poorly functioning kidney, i.e. with less than 10% of overall renal function, is often difficult. It is probably better to be conservative and perform a pyeloplasty in those children less than 1 year of age in the hope that there will be some recovery of renal function (King et al 1984).

All children under the age of 1 year should have a cystogram to exclude vesico-ureteric reflux. If reflux is found, a bladder catheter should be left in situ after the pyeloplasty to diminish the risk of an anastomotic leak.

SURGICAL TECHNIQUE

There are many different techniques available to repair a PUJ obstruction. The decision as to which type to use should be taken at the time of surgery after the PUJ has been exposed. The dismembered pyeloplasty (Anderson 1963) is suitable for the majority of patients. Occasionally there is a dependent PUJ with a fairly long narrow ureteric segment, and such a pyeloplasty may leave the surgeon short of ureteric length. A Culp pyeloplasty (Culp & De Weerd 1951) is then more suitable.

SURGICAL APPROACH

Three approaches may be used: the loin, the anterior extraperitoneal or the lumbotomy. All kidneys can be approached by the loin with excellent exposure, but it is a fairly painful incision postoperatively. The anterior extraperitoneal approach is excellent in younger children with a reasonably large renal pelvis, but access is more difficult in older or obese children. Its main advantage is speed of access and excellent postoperative healing of the scar. The lumbotomy incision is now coming back into fashion. Its proponents emphasize the relatively pain-free postoperative period, thus allowing early discharge from hospital. Whichever approach is favoured, it is important to stay extraperitoneal. Any tear in the peritoneum allows the small bowel to herniate through the defect and obscure the operative field. If bilateral PUJ obstructions are being dealt with, a transverse transperitoneal approach affords excellent exposure to both kidneys, but there is a significant risk of postoperative adhesions causing intestinal obstruction. I would therefore favour a bilateral anterior extraperitoneal approach which avoids the necessity of retowelling and repositioning of the patient. The following operative description applies to the loin approach.

DISMEMBERED PYELOPLASTY

The skin incision is made just below, and in line with, the twelfth rib. External and internal oblique muscles are divided by cutting diathermy, and the transversus abdominis is split at the line of its fibres. The peritoneum is gently pushed medially and a self-retaining Denis Browne ring retractor inserted.

The renal fascia is opened and the renal pelvis and PUJ are exposed using blunt and sharp dissection. In the majority of patients the PUJ is best approached anteriorly, but sometimes it is easier to rotate the kidney, retracting the lower pole forwards and upwards to approach the PUJ from behind. Full mobilization of the kidney with delivery into the wound is usually unnecessary.

The adventitia covering the renal pelvis and PUJ is incised laterally (Fig. 1.1). A 6/0 Dexon suture is placed in the ureter just below the narrowed segment. Further sutures are placed in the renal pelvis to mark the upper and lower margins of the proposed line of excision. The excess renal pelvis is resected. It should be trimmed with sharp scissors in a straight line without jagged margins. There is no evidence that radical trimming of the renal pelvis is necessary and it may lead to problems if the necks of the calyces are compromised. Therefore a moderate excision is all that is required. The upper ureter is divided just below the narrowed segment.

The adventitia of the upper 2–3 cm of the ureter is freed laterally (Fig. 1.2). The ureter is spatulated by incising its lateral margin, using fine sharp scissors, being careful to spare its medial blood supply. Normally a length of approximately 1–2 cm of spatulation is adequate.

The upper part of the renal pelvis is closed with a running 5/0 or 6/0 Dexon suture, until the length of opened renal pelvis equals the length of spatulated ureter.

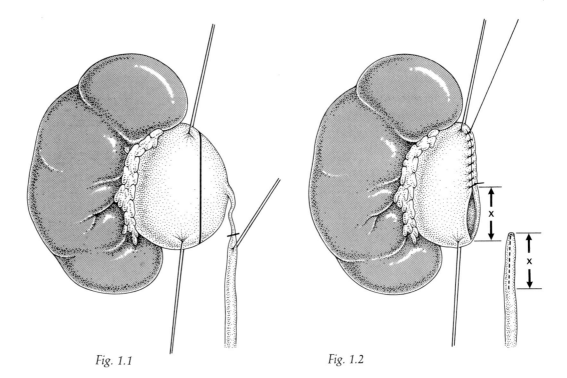

Fig. 1.1   *Fig. 1.2*

The ureter is anastomosed to the renal pelvis (Fig. 1.3). The first three sutures are of critical importance. The first stitch is an everting suture approximating the lower margin of the renal pelvis to the lower margin of the spatulated ureter (A). A further interrupted everting suture is then placed on each side of this initial stitch (B & C). The importance of these stitches lies in the fact that this is the narrowest part of the anastomosis.

The posterior aspect of the anastomosis is then completed using 6/0 Dexon (Fig. 1.4).

A fine catheter is passed temporarily through the anastomosis and the anterior closure is performed using another running 6/0 suture (Fig. 1.5). The fine catheter prevents the inadvertent picking up of the posterior wall during this final stage of the anastomosis. The catheter is removed just before the anastomosis is completed (Fig. 1.6).

If the ureteric length is too great to exactly fit into the opened renal pelvis, it is trimmed near its upper margin (Fig. 1.7). For infant pyeloplasties, optical magnification will be found helpful.

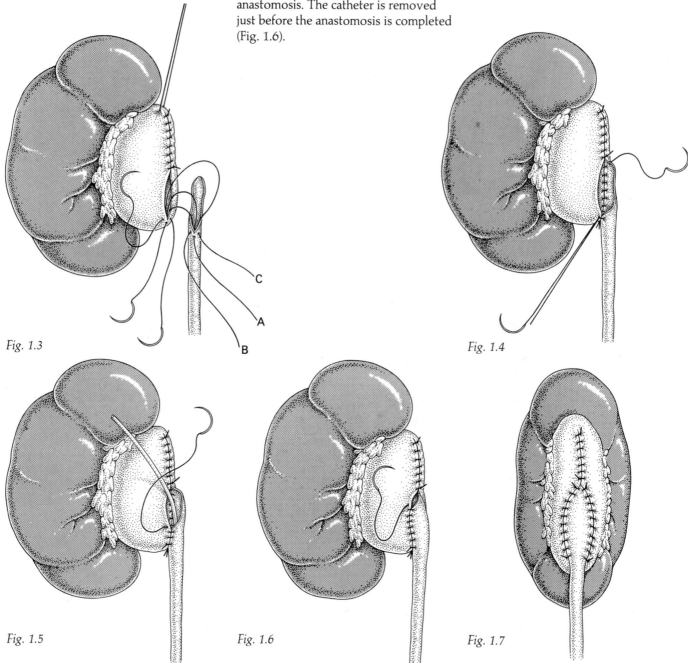

Fig. 1.3

Fig. 1.4

Fig. 1.5

Fig. 1.6

Fig. 1.7

Drainage

Normally no splint or nephrostomy catheter is used. If, for some reason, the anastomosis was technically difficult, the tissues are extremely soft and friable from recent infection, or the kidney is grossly hydronephrotic and baggy, the use of a nephrostomy and a ureteric splint is a reasonable safety precaution. A fine 4 or 6F splint is passed through a hydronephrotic calyx and down into the ureter. A nephrostomy is performed using a 12 or 14F Malécot catheter. A retroperitoneal corrugated drain is left in situ postoperatively.

THE CULP/DE WEERD PYELOPLASTY

Occasionally there is a shortage of ureteric length with a dependent type of PUJ obstruction. A dismembered pyeloplasty will then leave the surgeon in difficulties and in this situation a Culp pyeloplasty should be performed.

Exposure of the kidney is as before. The incision on the renal pelvis is carried from the mid-part of the renal pelvis superiorly, curving around and down the anterolateral margin of the upper ureter for approximately 1–2 cm (Fig. 1.8). The length of the flap and the length of the incision in the ureter must be equal. It is important that the base of the flap is of adequate width so that the length-to-width ratio is no more than three to one.

Whether the flap is fashioned in a longitudinal manner (Scardino 1967) or in a spiral fashion depends on the shape of the renal pelvis. A long renal pelvis allows a vertical flap to be formed whereas a more rectangular shaped pelvis is better suited to a spiral shaped flap (Fig. 1.9).

The flap is rotated inferiorly and sutured to the ureter (Fig. 1.10). The initial sutures—A, B and C—are as for a dismembered pyeloplasty. These sutures are placed to join the apex of the flap to the lower margin of the ureteric opening.

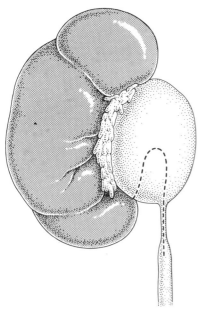

Fig. 1.8

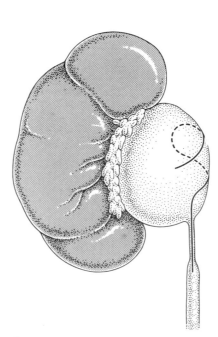

Fig. 1.9

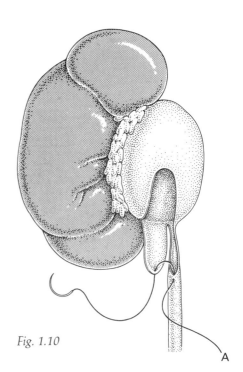

Fig. 1.10

A continuous 5/0 or 6/0 Dexon suture is then used to complete the anastomosis (Figs. 1.11, 1.12, 1.13). Again a ureteric splint is used temporarily to avoid picking up the posterior wall.

Drainage and postoperative management are the same as for a dismembered pyeloplasty.

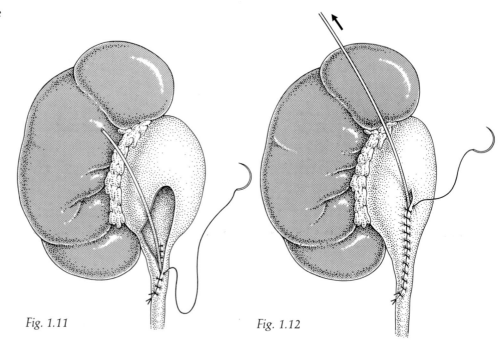

Fig. 1.11   Fig. 1.12

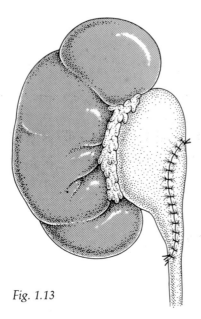

Fig. 1.13

LOWER POLE VESSELS

Sometimes a PUJ obstruction is associated with the presence of aberrant lower pole vessels. Whether these vessels are the cause of the obstruction or impinge on the PUJ secondarily is a matter of debate. When repairing an obstructed PUJ under these circumstances a dismembered type of pyeloplasty should be performed so that the vessels can be placed posterior to the anastomosis.

POSTOPERATIVE MANAGEMENT

The management of these patients varies, depending upon whether a nephrostomy tube and stent have been used. If neither is used, and there is no urinary leakage from the retroperitoneal drain, the latter can be removed on the fourth postoperative day and the child discharged home on the fifth day. If both a nephrostomy and a stent have been used, the stent is removed on the seventh postoperative day. A nephrostogram is performed routinely prior to removal of the nephrostomy tube, and provided this shows free drainage into the ureter, the tube is removed on the eighth day. Any urinary drainage will usually cease within 2 or 3 days.

In a review of 130 patients Homsy et al (1980) found that, with or without a urinary diversion, leakage of urine for 7 days postoperatively was compatible with a successful surgical result. If there is persistent urinary leakage, an obstruction at the site of the repair is likely. The passage of a retrograde catheter may open up such an obstructed anastomosis and the leakage will cease. If this conservative approach fails and leakage persists, re-exploration may be required. If the patient has a nephrostomy it is reasonable to send the child home with the nephrostomy catheter on free drainage and try clamping the catheter again at 1 month postoperatively. Hendren et al (1980) have reported using the nephrostomy track to fulgurate the oedematous tissue at the site of anastomosis with successful cessation of the urinary leakage.

Follow-up studies using either a DTPA renal scan or an intravenous urogram are performed at 3 months. Late complications of this operation are rare.

REFERENCES

Anderson J L 1963 Hydronephrosis. Heinemann, London
Culp O S, De Weerd J H 1951 A pelvic flap operation for certain types of
  ureteropelvic obstruction: observations after two years experience.
  Journal of Urology 71: 523–529
Hendren W H, Radhakrishnan J R, Middleton A W 1980 Pediatric
  pyeloplasty. Journal of Pediatric Surgery 15: 133–144
Homsy Y, Simard J, Debs C 1980 Pyeloplasty: to divert or not to divert?
  Urology 16: 577
King L R, Loughlin P W F, Block E C, Bowie J D, Gasony K, Hanna H K
  1984 The case for immediate pyeloplasty in the neonate with
  ureteropelvic junction obstruction. Journal of Urology 132: 725–728
Ransley P G, Manzoni G H 1985 Extended role of DTPA scan in assessing
  function and PUJ obstruction in neonates. Dialogues in Pediatric Urology
  8: 36–38
Scardino P L 1967 Uretero pelvic lesions. In: Bergman H (ed) The ureter.
  Hooper Medical Division, New York, p 508–526

Chapter 2

The surgery of upper urinary tract duplication

J. H. Johnston

Introduction

This chapter is concerned mainly with the techniques of upper and lower heminephrectomy and ureterectomy in cases of ureteric duplication. Conservational surgery avoiding heminephrectomy is also discussed, but vesico-ureteric reflux with double ureters, local management of ectopic ureterocele and pelvi-ureteric obstruction affecting the lower hemikidney are discussed elsewhere in the book.

UPPER HEMINEPHRECTOMY

The main indications for this operation are in the treatment of ectopic ureterocele and ectopic ureter when the upper hemikidney has been shown by radionuclide studies to be making no useful contribution to overall renal function.

The kidney is exposed by the surgeon's preferred method and is delivered into the wound. As a rule, because of pathological changes, the line of demarcation between the two hemikidneys is obvious on inspection and palpation. The vessels supplying the upper hemikidney are demonstrated by hilar dissection and divided between ligatures. If there is doubt concerning the distribution of an artery, it may be necessary to clamp it temporarily and observe the effect on the kidney tissue. Often there is an artery, of indeterminate origin, entering the apex of the kidney which must be ligated and divided. The renal capsule is incised above the demarcation line on the anterior and posterior aspects of the upper hemikidney and dissected downwards (Fig. 2.1); the redundant capsule is useful in the later closure of the upper extremity of the remaining lower hemikidney. When the upper hemikidney is dysplastic or severely scarred, it may not be possible to separate the renal capsule from it.

A sharp knife or scissors dissection is needed to separate the hemikidneys but the precise technique varies; often the plane between the two is irregular in three dimensions since the contiguous surfaces tend to be concavo-convex with the upper hemikidney sitting in the lower, like an egg in a egg-cup. It is therefore frequently advisable to divide the kidney erring on the diseased side, cutting into the calyces of the upper hemikidney and then trimming off these calyces and their related parenchyma secondarily. The optimal plane of division is closely into the lower hemikidney, preferably incising the tissue on either side of the exposed lower renal pelvis obliquely so as to facilitate closure (Fig. 2.2).

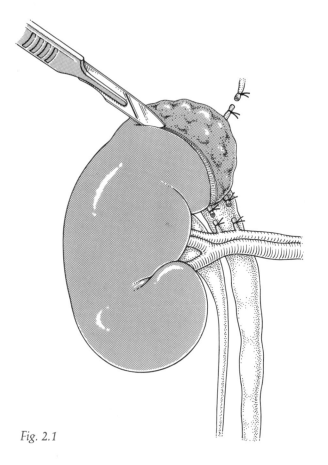

Fig. 2.1

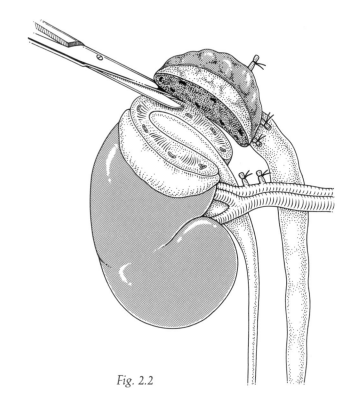

Fig. 2.2

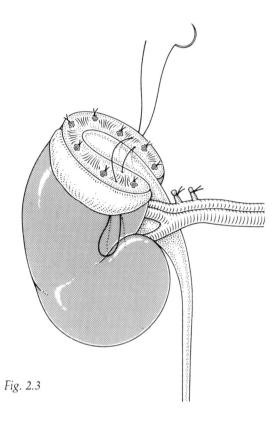

Fig. 2.3

Bleeding vessels on the cut renal surfaces are under-run and ligated with fine catgut sutures. Vertical mattress sutures of catgut are inserted, picking up the reflected capsule from the upper hemikidney in order to avoid the sutures cutting through (Fig. 2.3).

Tying the mattress sutures apposes the cut surfaces (Fig. 2.4). The hemikidney is now suspended by a narrow pedicle and, in order to avoid possible subsequent torsion, the renal capsule must be sutured to the adjacent musculo-fascial tissues on the posterior abdominal wall.

If closure of the upper pole of the lower hemikidney as described above proves to be impossible, the pole may, after the cut parenchymal vessels are controlled, be left open and the raw surfaces covered by suturing adjacent perirenal fat over them (Fig. 2.5).

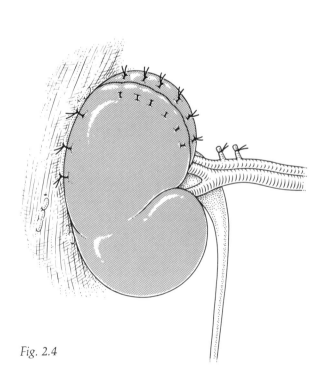

Fig. 2.4

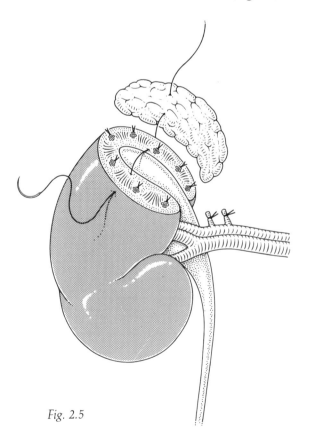

Fig. 2.5

URETERECTOMY FROM THE UPPER HEMIKIDNEY

When upper heminephrectomy has been performed as the definitive treatment of ectopic ureterocele or for the relief of urinary incontinence when an ectopic ureter opens on the vulva or vagina, the ureter need be excised only as low as can be obtained within the limits of the abdominal heminephrectomy incision. The same recommendations apply when an ectopic ureter opens into the urethra in either sex and there is no urethro-ureteric reflux. However, when urethro-ureteric reflux exists, incomplete urete-rectomy produces what is effectively a urethral diverticulum, which may lead to persistent urinary infection or even to calculus formation in the ureteric stump. Nevertheless, because of difficulties in operative exposure and the risk of harming the vesico-urethral sphincters and, in the male, the ejaculatory apparatus, it is often preferable to carry out an incomplete ureterectomy in the first instance and await events.

When excision of the stump of an ectopic ureter opening into the urethra or into a cystically dilated seminal vesicle proves to be essential, the preferred exposure is transvesical. Through a lower abdominal incision the bladder is opened via its anterior wall in routine fashion. A vertical incision is made through the vesico-trigonal wall midway between the ureteric orifices (Fig. 2.6).

The ureteric stump and, in the male, an involved seminal vesicle are readily mobilized to their terminations and excised (Fig. 2.7).

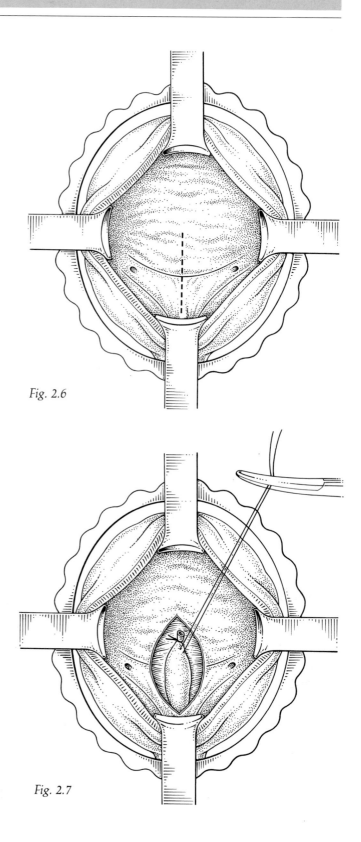

Fig. 2.6

Fig. 2.7

LOWER HEMINEPHRECTOMY

This procedure is less often required than upper heminephrectomy. It is indicated when vesico-ureteric reflux has produced irreparable destruction of the lower hemikidney while the upper moiety remains unaffected.

The technique (see Fig. 2.8) is essentially similar to that described for upper heminephrectomy, and it is again important to suture the renal capsule to the adjacent musculature in order to avoid the possibility of postoperative torsion.

URETERECTOMY FROM THE LOWER HEMIKIDNEY

Complete ureterectomy is needed here in order to avoid a refluxing ureteric stump which might allow persistent infection. A separate lower abdominal incision is required; an oblique, muscle-cutting incision in the iliac fossa, as described for megaureter (Chapter 5), is appropriate.

The blood supplies of the twin ureters are closely interrelated and careful dissection is needed to define, ligate and divide the vessels going to the ureter that is being removed in order to avoid endangering its fellow. Some one or two inches above the bladder, the two ureters fuse to share a common wall; attempts to separate them would almost certainly damage the ureter being retained. The refluxing ureter should be resected to and divided at the point of fusion; the stump is then laid open to the level of the bladder musculature, leaving the common wall intact. The resulting vesical aperture is closed with one or two catgut sutures (Fig. 2.9), care being taken to avoid occlusion or kinking of the remaining ureter. Redundant fringes from the incised ureteric stump may be excised but removal of its mucosa is not necessary. Drainage of the wound for a few days is advisable because temporary leakage from the bladder is possible.

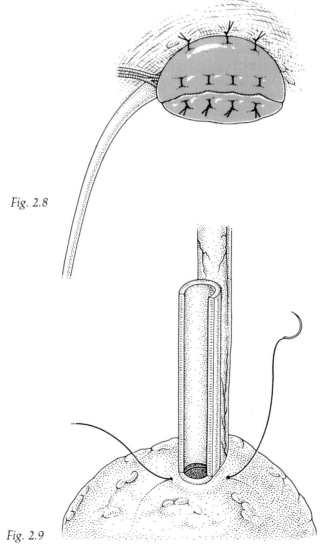

Fig. 2.8

Fig. 2.9

CONSERVATIONAL SURGERY IN CASES OF URETERIC DUPLICATION

Upper uretero-pyelostomy (Fig. 2.10)
This procedure is indicated as an alternative to upper heminephrectomy when the upper hemikidney is shown on intravenous urography and on radionuclide studies to possess useful function. The dilated ureter from the upper hemikidney is divided and anastomosed end to side to the pelvis of the lower hemikidney. Intralumenal drainage to the exterior is usually not needed but a soft drain should be left to the region of the anastomosis. The management of the lower ureter is as already discussed.

Lower pelvi-ureterostomy (Fig. 2.11)
This technique is applicable, as an alternative to heminephrectomy, in cases of reflux to the lower hemikidney when the parenchyma has sufficient function to be of overall value to the patient but anti-reflux surgery is considered inadvisable because the refluxing ureter is severely dilated. The pelvis of the lower hemikidney is divided and anastomosed end to side to the ureter draining the upper hemikidney. Since the latter is ordinarily a very narrow tube, meticulous suturing is essential in order to avoid its stenosis or devascularization. A transanastomotic splint brought to the exterior and nephrostomy drainage of the lower hemikidney are advisable. The lower end of the refluxing ureter is managed as discussed above.

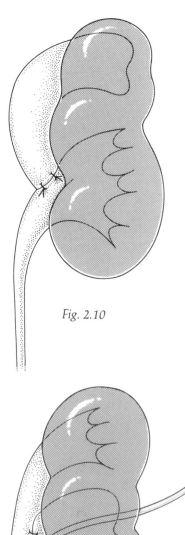

Fig. 2.10

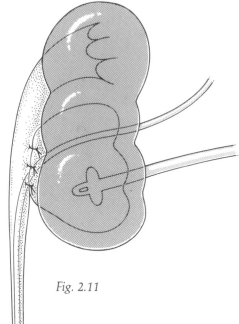

Fig. 2.11

Chapter 3

Excision of ectopic ureterocele

J. H. Johnston

Introduction

With a small ectopic ureterocele the urinary tract pathology is often restricted to the ureter and hemikidney drained by the ureterocele. In such cases decompression of the ureterocele by upper hemi-nephrectomy or, if the hemikidney shows useful function, by division of its ureter and anastomosis of the proximal end to the side of the pelvis of the lower hemikidney, often suffices (Johnston 1972). Occasionally, however, such management is ineffective; the de-functioned ureterocele and ureteric stump may fill with pus and require resection at a later date (Rickwood 1985, personal communication).

When a large ectopic ureterocele encroaches upon and obstructs the twin ureter or, less often, the contralateral ureter, or when it partially occludes the vesical outlet and interferes with bladder emptying, surgical excision of the ureterocele is often advisable as a primary procedure; otherwise it may by its bulk, even when empty of urine, continue to produce secondary obstructive effects if only a decompression procedure has been carried out.

Figure 3.1 illustrates a common anatomical arrangement in which the intravesical portion of the ureter draining the lower hemikidney is obstructed by being stretched over the surface of a large, tense ureterocele. If the ureterocele is decompressed and flabby, reflux may occur to the twin ureter.

SURGICAL TECHNIQUE

The ureterocele should be excised with reimplantation of the twin ureter into the bladder.

With the patient in the supine position, an oblique muscle-cutting incision is made in the iliac fossa (left in the drawing) to expose the double ureters extraperitoneally (Fig. 3.2).

The ureters are mobilized and the bladder is opened by an incision on its supero-lateral aspect to reveal the ectopic ureterocele with the orifice of the twin ureter on its surface (Fig. 3.3). For the purpose of clarity of illustration the orifice of the ureterocele is shown to be just proximal to the bladder neck; more often, as is discussed later, it is situated in the posterior urethra.

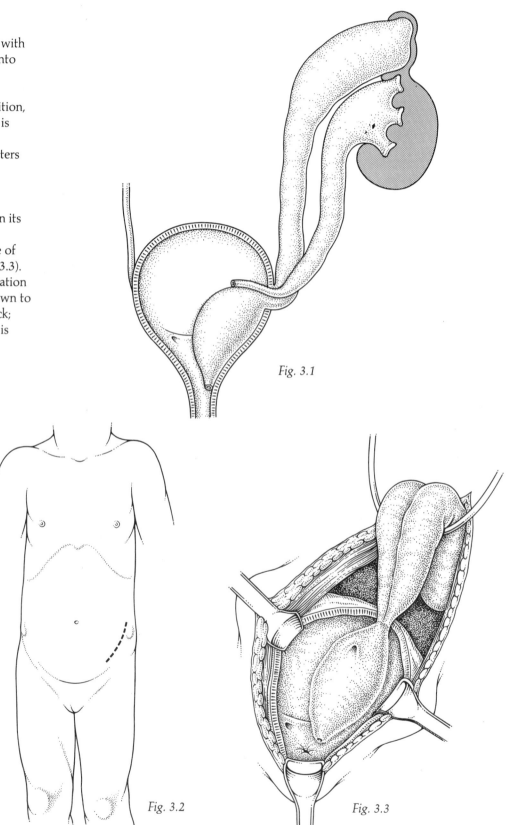

Fig. 3.1

Fig. 3.2

Fig. 3.3

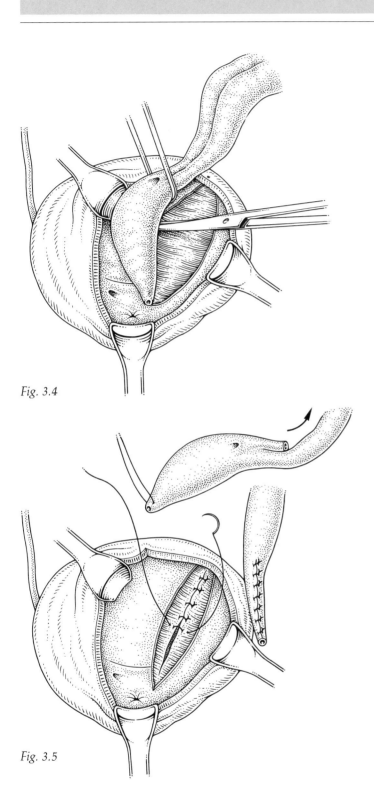

Fig. 3.4

Fig. 3.5

The bladder mucosa is incised around the margins of the ureterocele which is then dissected from the underlying musculature (Fig. 3.4).

The ureterocele and the twin ureter are mobilized from the bladder (Fig. 3.5). Since the detrusor muscle behind the ureterocele has been stretched and thinned, this area is reinforced by bringing in stronger muscle tissue from each side. Because the double ureters share a common wall near their termination, attempts to separate them by dissection would endanger the blood supply of the twin ureter. The latter must be divided above the level of ureteric fusion; it is usually sufficiently dilated to need operative trimming and narrowing prior to reimplantation to the bladder. (The technique is illustrated in Chapter 5 and is identical with that described for the obstructed megaureter.) The ureterocele and its ureter are freed towards the kidney.

The narrowed ureter from the lower hemikidney is implanted into the bladder to lie on the reinforced bed of the ureterocele (Fig. 3.6). The bladder mucosa on either side is mobilized sufficiently to allow it to be sutured over the ureter. The bladder is closed with tube drainage to the surface, and the abdominal muscle and cutaneous incisions are sutured.

There are now several management possibilities concerning the upper hemikidney and its ureter:

a.   Through a separate flank incision, after moving the patient to a lateral position on the operating table, upper heminephro-ureterectomy is indicated if, as is commonly the case, the upper hemikidney has shown no useful function on prior intravenous urography and DMSA scanning. Alternatively, if the upper hemikidney is worth preserving, its ureter is divided near its origin and a proximal end-to-side anastomosis is performed between it and the pelvis of the lower hemikidney. The distal portion of the ureter is excised.

b.   Through a stab incision near the flank, with the patient in only a slightly altered table position, temporary terminal cutaneous ureterostomy can be performed, with resection of the redundant ureter. This method is indicated under two circumstances: first, when excision of the ureterocele has been carried out in a sick, toxic, infected infant in whom further operative intervention is considered inadvisable; and second, when one is uncertain about the usefulness of the upper hemikidney so that measurement of the volume and

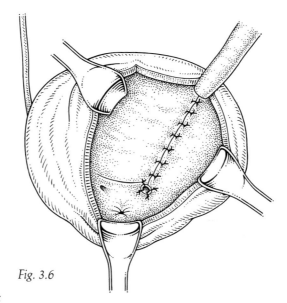

Fig. 3.6

quality of the urine drained from it may be valuable. Some 2–3 weeks later either of the possibilities listed under *a.* can be carried out.

COMMENT

When, as is commonly the case, an ectopic ureterocele extends into the proximal urethra, attempts at its total removal become a hazard to the urethral wall, with the possibility of stricture formation. In such circumstances it is preferable to excise only the intravesical portion of the ureterocele, as described above. The intraurethral extension is treated by de-roofing, leaving the ureterocele floor to form part of the lining of the urethra. It is important to avoid leaving behind portions of the ureterocele wall, which might cause a valvular type of urethral obstruction.

REFERENCES

Johnston J H 1972 Problems in the diagnosis and management of ectopic ureters and ureteroceles. In: Johnston J H, Scholtmeyer R J (eds) Problems in paediatric urology. Excerpta Medica, Amsterdam

Chapter 4

The surgical management of Wilms' tumour

J. D. Frank

Introduction

The management of childhood cancer changed dramatically with the advent of radiotherapy and, later, chemotherapy, and nowhere is this better demonstrated than in the treatment of patients with Wilms' tumour. Surgical treatment alone led to a survival of only 20%. The addition of the other treatment modalities has led to an overall survival of greater than 85%. Nephrectomy therefore plays only a part in the overall management of these patients, and before subjecting a a child to surgery it is necessary to answer three important questions:

1. Is the mass a Wilms' tumour? An incorrect diagnosis was made in 5% of patients in the National Wilms' Tumour Study (D'Angio et al 1976). Fourteen of the 30 incorrect diagnoses were for benign conditions.
2. Is the disease unilateral or bilateral?
3. Is there any evidence of tumour thrombus within the renal vein, inferior vena cava or right atrium?

PRESENTATION AND INVESTIGATIONS

The majority of children present with an abdominal mass, although pain and haematuria are the presenting features in 25% and fever associated with anorexia and vomiting in approximately 5%. There are a number of sophisticated tests available for the investigation of an abdominal mass but it is important that these answer specific questions without being over-invasive and exposing the child to unnecessary irradiation.

The initial investigation should be an ultrasound examination of the abdomen. This will confirm whether the lesion is solid or cystic. If solid, the inferior vena cava can be examined in detail to exclude the presence of tumour thrombus within its lumen. If the vena cava is compressed by the weight of the tumour, examination may be repeated in the prone position using slings. Routine investigations should include the blood pressure, a 24-hour urine collection for vanillylmandelic acid and a chest X-ray to exclude metastases.

The intravenous urogram remains a useful investigation. The diagnosis of a Wilms' tumour is confirmed by the characteristic distortion and displacement of the renal collecting system or by non-function of the affected side. This study can be combined with an inferior caval venogram by injecting the contrast medium via a leg vein and taking early rapid sequential pictures of the inferior vena cava. Tumour thrombus may occasionally be noted on this examination which has been previously missed by ultrasound. If the ultrasound examination or the venogram shows tumour to be present within the inferior vena cava, its upper limit must be clearly defined. The ultrasound examination will ordinarily show this,

but if there is any suspicion that the tumour is extending into the right atrium, echocardiography should be performed. If atrial tumour is confirmed, a right heart catheterization is then carried out to define the extent and size of the tumour thrombus.

Computed tomography may be helpful in two situations: a suspicious but not diagnostic lesion on the chest X-ray can be further elucidated, and the presence of a metastasis can be confirmed or refuted. Suspicious areas in the contralateral kidney on the intravenous urogram may also be defined in more detail. Arteriography is rarely necessary in the diagnosis of a Wilms' tumour. It occasionally helps in planning the surgical approach for a pretreated patient with bilateral tumours or in the surgery of a Wilms' tumour in a horseshoe kidney.

SURGICAL MANAGEMENT

The surgical management of a patient with a Wilms' tumour will be influenced by the size of the tumour, the presence of metastases, the presence of thrombus within the inferior vena cava or right atrium and evidence of bilateral disease. The traditional teaching of tumour surgery has been that a tumour should be excised if possible. Wilms' tumours, however, are normally extremely sensitive to both chemotherapy and radiotherapy, and therefore there are a number of indications for pretreatment of a tumour prior to surgery. These are:

1. *If the tumour is extremely large and it is thought that excision would be technically difficult.* It is then wiser to carry out a needle biopsy to confirm the diagnosis and pretreat such a patient prior to performing a nephrectomy. These large tumours rapidly shrink in size, and safe and relatively easy surgery may then be performed. The days of heroic surgery

which puts the patient's life at risk are over.

2. *The presence of extensive inferior vena caval or right atrial tumour thrombus.* If tumour thrombus is found to extend into the inferior vena cava but end below the diaphragm, it is reasonable to proceed to a nephrectomy with removal of the tumour thrombus from the inferior vena cava. If, however, there is extension of the thrombus above the diaphragm or into the right atrium, the patient may either be pretreated or the tumour together with the thrombus may be removed by using right heart by-pass surgery. There have been many reports in the literature of successful surgery using this latter technique (Gonzalez et al 1983). However, there have also been reports of successful pretreatment of such patients with chemotherapy and radiotherapy (Kogan et al 1986) and I would favour this more conservative approach. What must be avoided at all costs is an attempt to remove intravascular thrombus without adequate proximal and distal vascular control. Tumour embolization under such conditions can lead to an operative death. The National Wilms' Tumour Study (NWTS) trial showed that the presence of tumour within the renal vein or inferior vena cava did not adversely affect the survival of 37 patients (Leape et al 1978).

Bilateral Wilms' tumours

At least 4% of patients with Wilms' tumours will have bilateral disease and in more than one-third of these patients bilaterality is not suspected preoperatively. Thus, when carrying out a laparotomy for a Wilms' tumour, the apparently normal kidney should be examined first as the presence of bilateral disease will influence further surgical management. The majority of patients in the past with bilateral disease have undergone nephrectomy of the kidney with major tumour involvement together with excision biopsy or partial nephrectomy of the contralateral less-involved side. Total excision of the tumour is usually not possible, and in 75% of children with bilateral disease, residual tumour will be left behind in spite of repeated surgical procedures. The 2-year survival rate, however, is extremely good at 87% overall or 83% of those patients left with residual disease (Kay 1985). These tumours occur in a young age group and there is often nephroblastomatosis present in both kidneys. The principles of treatment have now been modified so that the surgical subcommittee of NWTS suggests that the aim of therapy should be to preserve as much functioning renal parenchyma as possible by adequate treatment of the tumour, through repeated resections if necessary, but avoiding nephrectomy until all conservative measures fail (Kelalis 1985). At the initial transperitoneal exploration, suspicious areas should be biopsied and lymph nodes sampled so that accurate staging can be undertaken and appropriate treatment planned. Conservative treatment is then continued for as long as there is an objective response, as noted by ultrasound and/or CT scans. If there is no response or less than 50% reduction of tumour size, a second-look laparotomy is performed at the end of 3 months. This laparotomy has the intention of maximum conservation of renal parenchyma with either a partial nephrectomy or excision biopsy of the tumour. If all the tumour is removed, chemotherapy is continued according to stage and no radiotherapy is given. If nephrectomy seems inevitable, definitive surgery is deferred, a re-biopsy is performed and chemotherapy and radiotherapy are given. At a suitable time, depending on the continued shrinkage of the tumour but at not less than 6 months, a third-look laparotomy is performed and definitive surgery is carried out. Apart from the surgical management of these patients, appropriate radiotherapy and chemotherapy are given depending upon the stage (see Table 4.1).

Table 4.1 Current staging of Wilms' tumour (NWTS-3)

Stage I
Tumour limited to kidney, completely excised. Capsular surface intact; no tumour rupture; no residual tumour apparent beyond margins of resection.

Stage II
Tumour extends beyond kidney but is completely excised. Regional extension of tumour; vessel infiltration; tumour biopsied or local spillage of tumour confined to the flank. No residual tumour apparent at or beyond margins of excision.

Stage III
Residual non-haematogenous tumour confined to the abdomen. Lymph node involvement of hilus, peri-aortic chains or beyond; diffuse peritoneal contamination by tumour spillage or peritoneal implants of tumour; tumour extends beyond surgical margins either microscopically or macroscopically; tumour not completely removable because of local infiltration into vital structures.

Stage IV
Tumour deposits beyond stage III, i.e. lung, liver, bone, brain.

Stage V
Bilateral renal involvement at diagnosis.

SURGICAL TECHNIQUE

The aims of surgery therefore are:
1. An initial examination of the apparently normal kidney to exclude bilateral disease;
2. Early ligation of the renal artery and vein prior to extensive mobilization of the kidney;
3. Nephrectomy without capsular breach.

The procedure
The patient is placed in the supine position and an extensive transverse, upper abdominal, muscle-cutting incision is made (Fig. 4.1). The peritoneum is opened, the liver is inspected for metastases, and the colon over the apparently normal kidney is reflected medially.

The renal fascia is then incised and the anterior and posterior surfaces of the kidney are carefully inspected (Fig. 4.2). If the kidney is tumour free, a contralateral nephrectomy is then undertaken. If tumour is found, a biopsy is taken and management undertaken using the bilateral Wilms' tumour protocol.

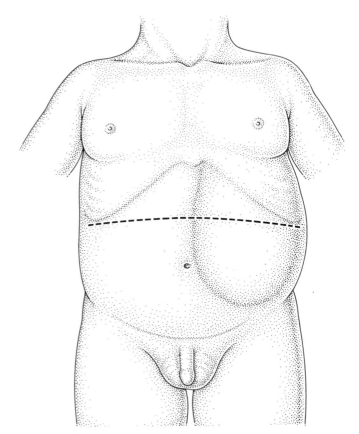

Fig. 4.1

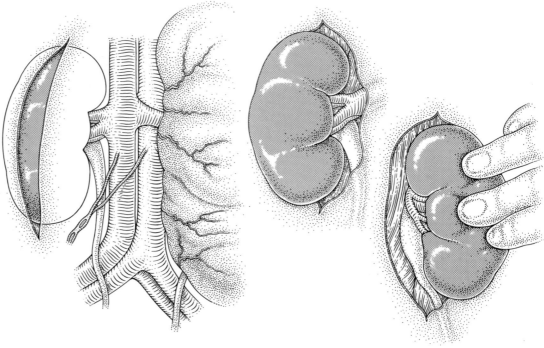

Fig. 4.2

The colon on the side of the tumour is mobilized medially by incising the lateral peritoneum (Fig. 4.3). If there is tumour invasion of the meso-colon or the colon, they should be left attached to the tumour and excised in continuity.

The ureter and gonadal vessels are identified as they pass over the pelvic brim and are ligated and divided separately (Fig. 4.4).

The ureter is lifted up and a plane is developed behind the ureter. The dissection is then carried out with sharp dissection along the aorta so that the lymph nodes are taken along with the specimen (Fig. 4.5).

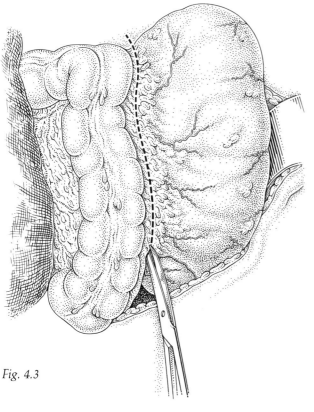

Fig. 4.3

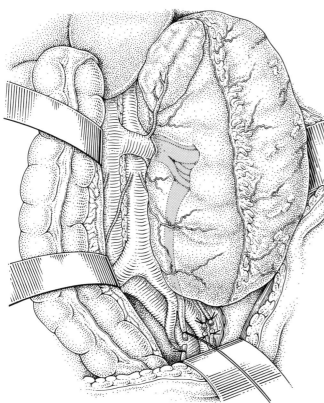

Fig. 4.4

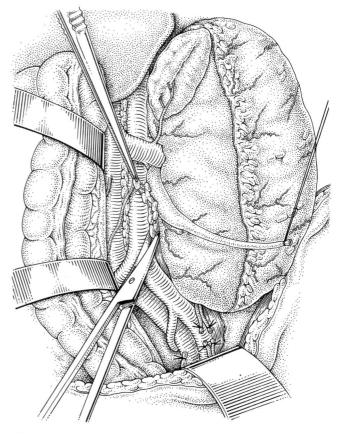

Fig. 4.5

When the renal pedicle is reached the vein overlies the artery. The vein is palpated to exclude the presence of tumour thrombus within it. Provided it is clear, division of the artery and vein can then be undertaken (Figs 4.6, 4.7). It is preferable to ligate the artery first, but occasionally with an extremely large tumour it is difficult to visualize the artery because it lies posterior to the vein. Under these circumstances the vein may be divided first. Care, however, must be taken because venous congestion of the tumour will occur and there is a danger of capsular rupture. Normally a sling can be passed around the vein and it can be lifted either superiorly or inferiorly out of the way of the artery, allowing the latter to be ligated and divided. The para-aortic lymph nodes, together with surrounding tissue, are then dissected off the aorta and inferior vena cava and removed with the kidney. If preoperative investigations have shown that there is tumour present within the inferior vena cava, adequate control of the cava must be obtained.

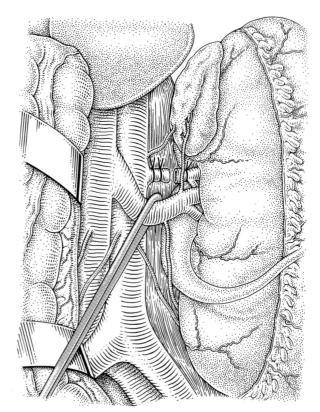

Fig. 4.6

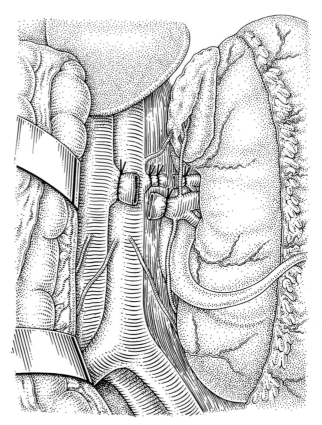

Fig. 4.7

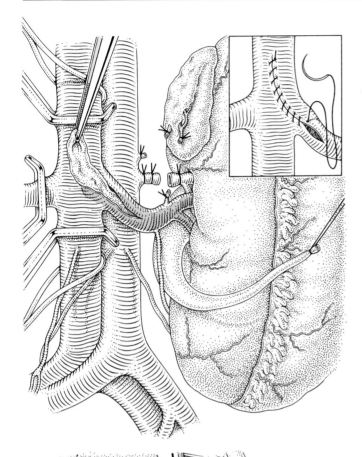

Fig. 4.8

Slings are placed around the inferior vena cava above and below the tumour thrombus. Both renal veins are also slung and the inferior vena cava is opened and the tumour removed (Fig. 4.8). The inferior vena cava is closed with 6/0 continuous silk or prolene sutures.

On the left side the lieno-renal ligament is divided. The adrenal gland is excised together with an upper pole tumour (Fig. 4.9) but may be left behind if the tumour is in the middle or lower poles. Care must be taken when removing the adrenal gland to ligate carefully the adrenal veins entering the inferior vena cava.

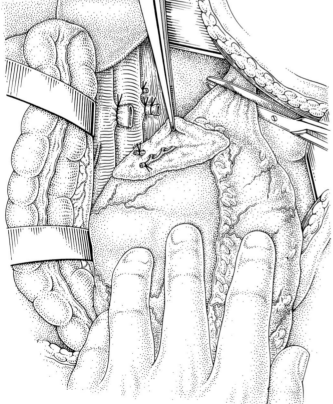

Fig. 4.9

The tumour is removed from the posterior abdominal wall using a sharp and a blunt dissection (Fig. 4.10). Haemostasis is obtained. No drainage is required. Postoperatively, continuous nasogastric suction with appropriate intravenous fluid therapy is given. Chemotherapy may start that evening or on the following day.

If there is local tumour invasion of structures that can be excised safely together with the tumour, this should be performed. Occasionally, however, invasion occurs that is surgically difficult to remove. Under these circumstances biopsies should be performed and chemotherapy given with a view to carrying out a second-look laparotomy, after appropriate treatment.

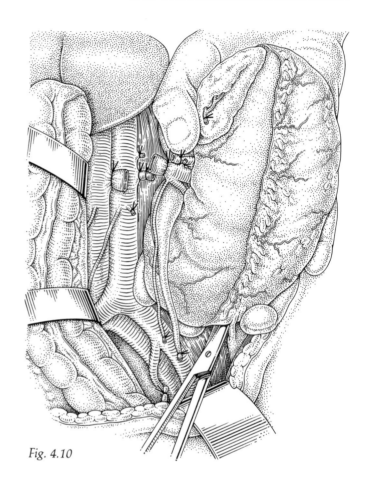

Fig. 4.10

REFERENCES

D'Angio G J, Evans A E, Breslow N et al 1976 The treatment of Wilms' tumour. Results of the National Wilms' Tumour Study. Cancer 38: 633–646

Gonzalez R, Clayman R V, Sheldon C A 1983 Management of intravascular nephroblastoma to avoid complications. Urological Clinics of North America 10: 407–415

Kay R 1985 Bilateral Wilms' tumor. Dialogues in Pediatric Urology 8 (10): 2

Kelalis P P 1985 Bilateral Wilms' tumour; surgical treatment. NWTS recommendations. Dialogues in Pediatric Urology 8 (10): 6–7

Kogan S J, Marans H, Santorineau M, Schneider K, Reda E, Levitt S B 1986 Successful treatment of renal vein and vena caval extension of nephroblastoma by preoperative chemotherapy. Journal of Urology 136: 312–319

Leape L L, Breslow N E, Bishop H C 1978 The surgical treatment of Wilms' tumour. Results of the National Wilms' Tumour Study. Annals of Surgery 187: 356–363

Chapter 5

Ureteric tailoring and reimplantation for uretero-vesical obstruction

J. H. Johnston

INDICATIONS

The technique described is particularly applicable to the obstructed megaureter. In this condition, which is most commonly unilateral, left-sided and affecting the male, there is a functional interference with the transmission of peristalsis in the terminal ureter. The obstructive ureteric segment remains of normal calibre while the ureter above becomes dilated, lengthened and tortuous, and the kidney shows hydronephrotic changes. The operative procedure can also be employed when there is a fibrotic uretero-vesical obstruction secondary to such infravesical obstructions as posterior urethral valves. The orthotopic ureterocele may be similarly managed, usually combined with excision of the ureterocele. The object of the operation is to relieve obstructive effects on the renal parenchyma, the consequences of which are commonly exacerbated by infection or by stone formation in the dilated system; at the same time subsequent vesico-ureteric reflux must be prevented.

PREOPERATIVE MEASURES

Infrequently, in the acutely obstructed case or when there is severe infection, preliminary drainage of the system is needed. This can usually be obtained by percutaneous insertion of a catheter into the renal pelvis under ultrasonographic guidance.

SURGICAL TECHNIQUE

An oblique, muscle-cutting incision is made in the appropriate iliac fossa, centred on the anterior superior iliac spine (Fig. 5.1). The dilated, tortuous ureter (left in the illustration) is exposed extraperitoneally.

The ureter is divided at the entrance to the bladder, with ligature of its distal extremity, and is straightened by the release of tortuosity as far as the ureteric blood supply allows (Fig. 5.2). The resulting redundant portion of the ureter is excised.

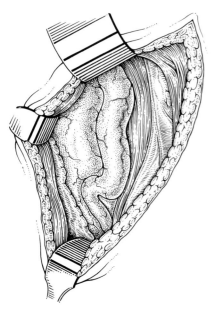

Fig. 5.1

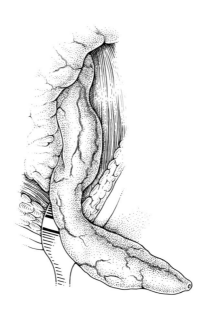

Fig. 5.2

The lowest 2–3 inches of the remaining ureter generally needs to be narrowed. This is best performed by passing a 10F catheter into the ureter. The catheter is then enclosed, through the ureteric wall, by Babcock or Hendren forceps (Fig. 5.3a). The ureter outside the grasping forceps is resected (Fig. 5.3b). It is important that the excised wedge of ureteral wall should be from its 'anti-mesenteric' aspect so that the mainly longitudinally running blood vessels will be preserved.

The narrowed segment of ureter is closed, using interrupted 4/0 catgut sutures (Fig. 5.4). The temptation to produce a normal ureteric calibre must be resisted so as to avoid jeopardizing the blood supply. There is no need for extensive ureteric remodelling; only that portion which is to form the new intravesical ureter need be narrowed.

The bladder is opened through an oblique incision on its supero-lateral aspect and a submucosal tunnel is fashioned between the incision and the region of the original ureteric orifice (Fig. 5.5). In order to avoid subsequent angulation of the ureter at the new vesical hiatus during bladder filling, the musculature at the mouth of the tunnel is sutured, with three catgut stitches, to the psoas muscle lateral to the external iliac vessels.

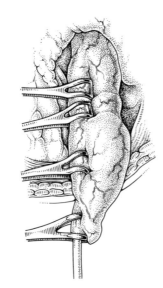

Fig. 5.3a

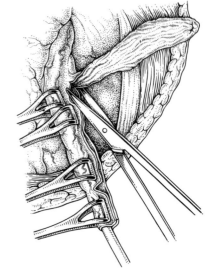

Fig. 5.3b

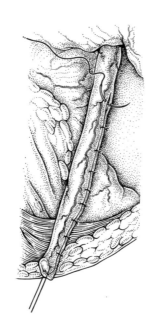

Fig. 5.4

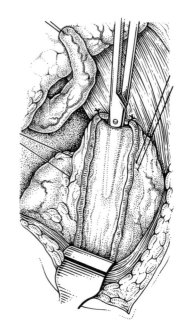

Fig. 5.5

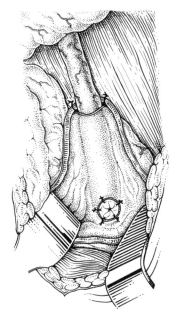

Fig. 5.6

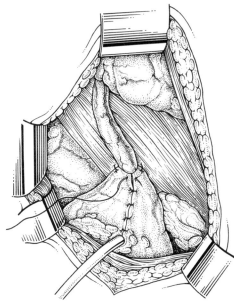

Fig. 5.7

The narrowed segment of ureter is passed through the submucosal tunnel and its extremity is sutured posteriorly to the bladder musculature and circumferentially to the mucosal edges of the tunnel (Fig. 5.6). One should aim at having the length of the new intravesical ureter five times its width. Ureteric splinting may or may not be considered necessary.

The bladder is closed with suprapubic drainage and the wound is sutured (Fig. 5.7).

COMMENTS AND RESULTS

Angulations of the ureter commonly exist in a tortuous megaureter but they are not, themselves, obstructive, and any which remain after the re-implantation operation straighten spontaneously with growth of the patient. However, secondary kinking at the pelvi-ureteric junction can persist and may necessitate pelvi-ureteroplasty.

The technique described can be relied upon to give highly satisfactory results, especially in cases of obstructed megaureter where kidney function is generally well preserved and ureteric peristalsis remains active or at least recoverable, in spite of complications. The psoas hitch procedure cannot be performed bilaterally. When both ureters require reimplantation, this aspect of the technique must be omitted or, alternatively, one ureter may be re-implanted as described and the other divided near the bladder, brought to the contralateral side retroperitoneally and anastomosed end to side to the re-implanted ureter.

Chapter 6

Temporary urinary diversion

J. H. Johnston

Introduction

Temporary urinary diversion during childhood may be achieved by catheters or by non-intubated methods. The choice depends partly on the pathology involved and partly on the expected duration of the required drainage.

INTUBATED DIVERSION

Catheter or tube drainage is commonly employed after reconstruction operations on the urinary tract or the genitalia. As a preliminary to surgery it is less often needed. However, per-urethral catheter drainage of the bladder may be indicated in the boy with urethral valves when the bladder is tensely distended and when correction of infection, dehydration or acidaemia is required prior to endoscopic valve fulguration. Suprapubic cystostomy is less often needed but can be obtained by percutaneous insertion of a polyethylene catheter if urethral catheterization fails.

Tube nephrostomy or pyelostomy may be wanted prior to definitive surgery for upper urinary tract obstruction, especially if there is an acute on chronic situation and if there is complicating infection. Also, preliminary drainage can be of prognostic value, by showing the volume and quality of the urine drained, in the decision as to whether or not a kidney is worth preserving. As a rule, percutaneous insertion of the polythene catheter under ultrasonic guidance presents little difficulty so that tube nephrostomy by open surgery is now seldom required. Nephrostomy catheters have been specifically designed for paediatric and neonatal use. If the duration of intubated kidney drainage exceeds 2–3 weeks, invasive infection is likely to ensue and endanger renal function. It is therefore advisable to proceed promptly either to the appropriate corrective surgery or to a non-intubated diversionary method.

NON-INTUBATED DIVERSION

Loop cutaneous ureterostomy

Temporary bilateral cutaneous loop ureterostomies provide, in appropriate cases, an easily performed and readily reversible means of lengthy tubeless drainage of the upper urinary tract. The main application of the method is in the infant boy with obstructive posterior urethral valves in whom, after the valves have been destroyed and the bladder is emptying readily, urinary stasis with damaging infection persists in the dilated, decompensated renal pelves and ureters. High external diversion then provides free, lengthy, kidney drainage while decompression of the systems below the stomas allows the upper urinary tract musculature to recover its tone and peristaltic activity.

Similar circumstances indicating the need for temporary ureterostomy may exist with other obstructive lesions, either supra- or infravesical, but it should be emphasized that the method is infrequently indicated. It has been much over-used since its first description (Johnston 1963). With modern developments in paediatric nephrology concerning the medical management of the infant with renal in-sufficiency due to obstructive uropathy, the indications are now exceptional and the use of the method should be limited to the circumstances indicated above and then only when the ureters are sufficiently dilated and tortuous to come readily to the abdominal surface.

Loop ureterostomy is illustrated diagrammatically in Figure 6.1.

Surgical technique. With the child under general anaesthesia in the lateral position, a short oblique incision is made just below the twelfth rib (Fig. 6.2). It is important that the ureteric stoma is fashioned in the flank; this allows the most direct drainage of the kidney and also leaves the entire lower ureter undisturbed in order to facilitate subsequent ureteric surgery which is occasionally needed to relieve uretero-vesical obstruction.

The dilated, elongated ureter is mobilized and brought to the surface, and the lumen is opened by a longitudinal incision (Fig. 6.3).

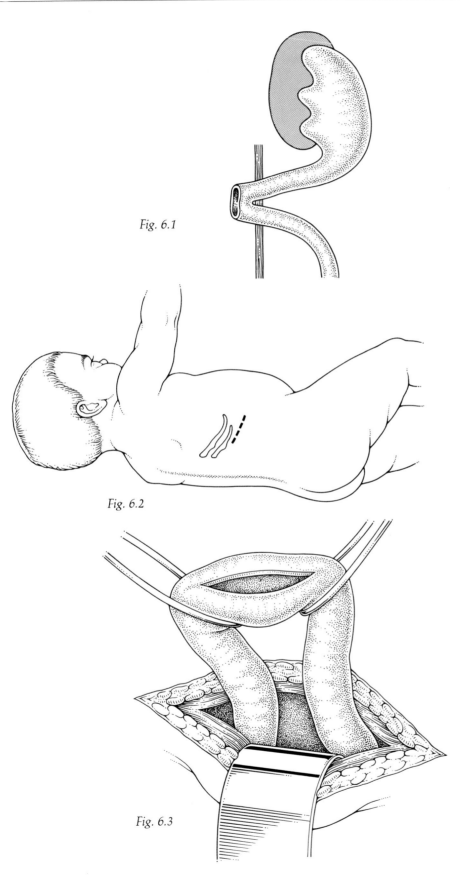

Fig. 6.1

Fig. 6.2

Fig. 6.3

The abdominal musculature is closed on either side of, and behind, the emerging loop of ureter (Fig. 6.4).

The margins of the ureteric incision are sutured to the skin edges, employing catgut or Dexon, to produce a double-barrelled stoma (Fig. 6.5).

Contralateral ureterostomy is performed in identical fashion when bilateral drainage is needed.

Ureterostomy drainage may be needed for weeks or months. If, when the child is thriving, the kidneys show useful function, descending ureterography under fluoroscopy shows effective peristalsis with free emptying to the bladder, and cystography demonstrates satisfactory bladder evacuation following micturition, the ureterostomies can be closed, one side at a time. During closure, the ureter is dissected from the abdominal parietes, and as a rule, redundant ureter has to be resected. An obliquely cut end-to-end anastomosis is performed; T-tube drainage to the exterior is advisable until healing is complete.

If, as is not uncommon in valve cases requiring ureterostomies, one kidney shows non function, nephrectomy is indicated. If descending ureterography reveals a lower ureteric obstruction due to fibrous replacement of the musculature of the intravesical segment, uretero-vesical reimplantation is needed prior to ureterostomy closure.

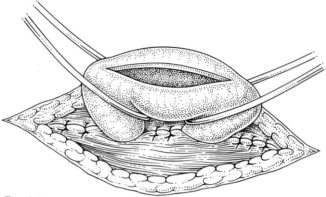

Fig. 6.4

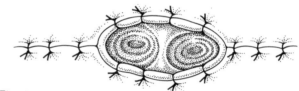

Fig. 6.5

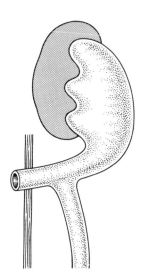

Fig. 6.6

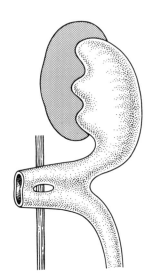

Fig. 6.7

Modification of the loop ureterostomy. Total defunctioning of the bladder by loop ureterostomy may be followed by vesical dysfunction, as revealed by cystography, even in the absence of any residual infravesical obstruction. As a rule, the problem is temporary and responds to a period of bladder re-education before the ureterostomies are closed; this can be achieved by inserting a Foley catheter into one of the lower ostomy stomas, inflating the balloon sufficiently to occlude the ureteric lumen, and then dripping saline from an intravenous set down to the bladder.

Infrequently, very lengthy diversion from a trabeculated bladder, especially if there has been severe infection, may lead to vesical contracture, and it may then not be possible to restore normal bladder function. In order to avoid this problem some authors have modified the original loop ureterostomy by forming a Y-anastomosis, as shown in Figure 6.6 (Sober 1972), or by a side-to-side anastomosis between the two ureterostomy limbs, as shown in Figure 6.7 (Williams & Cromie 1975), in order to allow some urine to continue to reach the bladder. Closure of such ureterostomies involves excision of the ureter distal to the uretero-ureteric anastomosis and suture of the resulting aperture in the ureteric wall.

Complications. Complications of loop ureterostomy and its modifications are encountered mainly in patients in whom the operation has been performed in-advisedly. It must be stressed that its safe performance requires that the ureters are markedly dilated and sufficiently lengthened and tortuous to allow them to come easily to the body surface. When the ureters do not fulfil these criteria, stomal retraction and stenosis may occur or ureteric de-vascularization may result, even to the degree of total ischaemic necrosis of the lower ureter.

CUTANEOUS VESICOSTOMY

This method of diversion is of value mainly as a temporizing measure in the infant with congenital neuropathy due to spinal dysraphism in whom the bladder is not emptying spontaneously and is not easily expressible manually so that the upper urinary tract is becoming dilated and renal function is threatened. Since the procedure is easily reversible there is the possibility of later closing the stoma and managing the bladder dysfunction conservatively when the patient reaches the age at which urinary control becomes important.

Surgical technique
A curved transverse incision is made rather higher than midway between the pubis and the umbilicus (Fig. 6.8). The skin and subcutaneous tissues are dissected proximally and distally from the aponeurosis and the linea alba is incised longitudinally.

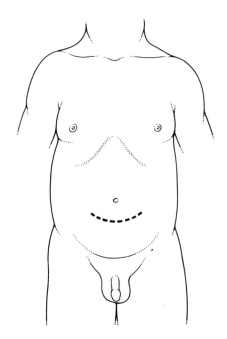

Fig. 6.8

The bladder is mobilized and opened by a small diathermy incision between holding sutures at the fundus (Fig. 6.9).

The aponeurosis is sutured with catgut to the bladder musculature around the stoma (Fig. 6.10).

The edges of the bladder stoma are sutured to the skin edges and the incision is closed on either side (Fig. 6.11).

Since the operation is performed only as a temporary procedure in infants in nappies, a urinary collecting appliance is not needed.

Complications. The main complications of cutaneous vesicostomy are stomal stenosis and bladder prolapse. The former is avoidable by ensuring that the bladder is sufficiently mobilized to come freely to the skin surface. The latter can be prevented by utilizing the bladder fundus for the vesicostomy and by fashioning a final cutaneous stoma no larger than that allowing the passage of a 25 Ch catheter (Duckett 1974).

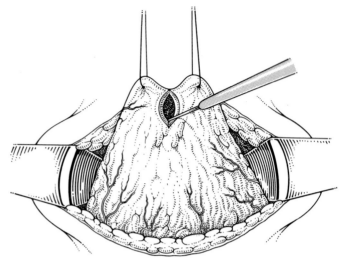

Fig. 6.9

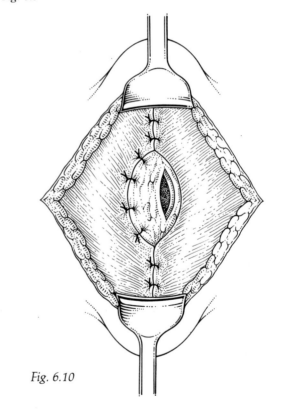

Fig. 6.10

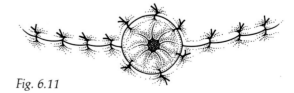

Fig. 6.11

REFERENCES

Duckett J W 1974 Cutaneous vesicostomy in childhood: the Blocksom technique. Urological Clinics of North America 1: 485
Johnston J H 1963 Temporary cutaneous ureterostomy in the management of advanced congenital urinary obstruction. Archives of Disease in Childhood 38: 161
Sober I 1972 Pelviureterostomy-en-Y. Journal of Urology 107: 473
Williams D I, Cromie W J 1975 Ring ureterostomy. British Journal of Urology 47: 789

Chapter 7

Permanent urinary diversion

A. M. K. Rickwood

INDICATIONS

Permanent urinary diversion is no longer commonly performed in children. Continuing indications are:

a. For patients with congenital neuropathic bladder, usually those with other major disabilities, in whom a more conservative approach has failed or is unrealistic. Those obliged to rely on a penile appliance or indwelling urethral catheter to stay dry may consider an abdominal urinary stoma a preferable alternative. Diversion is only occasionally the best means of dealing with secondary upper renal tract complications.
b. For patients with bladder exstrophy (and, rarely, epispadias) where the bladder is either too small for primary repair or where, following repair, further attempts to produce a continent bladder are unlikely to be rewarded.
c. For the occasional patient with pelvic malignancy requiring anterior exenteration.
d. For a few patients with miscellaneous conditions causing a combination of upper tract stasis and deteriorating renal function for whom it is felt that diversion offers the best prospect of materially delaying the onset of renal failure.

CHOICE OF DIVERSION

Intestinal conduit

This can be adapted to almost any situation; the conduit can be constructed from small or large bowel and the ureterointestinal anastomosis made refluxing or non-refluxing. The long-term results of refluxing conduits are poor (Middleton & Hendren 1976), with a formidable incidence of upper tract complications, some with an identifiable and remediable cause (e.g. stomal stenosis), and others without. Non-refluxing colonic conduits give superior, if not ideal, results (Althausen et al 1978) and should be regarded as the abdominal wall diversion of choice provided that colon is available and the ureters are neither massively dilated nor aperistaltic.

Terminal ureterostomy

At least one ureter must be chronically dilated to a diameter of 1 cm or more. Acutely dilated ureters have tenuous vascularity and are not suitable for ureterostomy. The procedure is straight-forward and largely eliminates the risk of gastrointestinal tract complications. In the medium term the results are generally superior to those obtained by refluxing conduits, but this advantage is lost in the long term.

Ureterosigmoidostomy in continuity

This requires good anal control and normal (or near normal) upper renal tracts. While superior technique and improved surveillance have largely eliminated previous problems of ascending infection and electrolyte imbalance, there remains considerable long-term risk of developing juxta-anastomotic colonic carcinoma (Stewart 1986), and patients undergoing this procedure require regular colonoscopy.

PREOPERATIVE MEASURES

The state of the upper renal tracts should be documented by an intra-venous urogram supplemented by isotope renography if there is evidence of renal parenchymal damage.

The stoma site is chosen in liaison with a stoma therapist. Normally this poses no difficulty provided that it is placed away from bony prominences and in an area free of skin creases both sitting and standing, but patients with spina bifida need extra care because of their tendency to develop spinal deformities. Here the stoma should be on the convex aspect of any scoliosis, while an upper abdominal site is preferable in the presence of lordosis. Sometimes there is *no* satisfactory site in children with severe and complex deformities.

Anal continence must be assessed in patients considered for ureterosigmoidostomy in continuity; the ability to retain 150–300 ml (depending on age) of lukewarm saline in the rectum for an hour or more is usually sufficient evidence that this is adequate.

Patients undergoing colonic conduit or ureterosigmoidostomy require bowel preparation. Combined enemas and saline bowel washouts are administered three times daily for 3 days along with low-residue diet for 2 days and clear fluids only for the third day. Neomycin and metronidazole are prescribed for 24 hours preoperatively.

SURGICAL TECHNIQUE

Abdominal incision and mobilization of ureters (Fig. 7.1)

The initial dissection is common to most diversions. A transverse lower abdominal incision (inset) is preferred for routine cases; in young, thin patients adequate access is obtained through a high Pfannenstiel incision, while in other cases the recti are divided transversely. A paramedian incision on the side opposite the intended stoma is advisable if difficulties are anticipated in gaining access to the ureters or in constructing a conduit. A Denis Browne ring retractor is inserted after opening the peritoneum, the patient tilted slightly head downwards, and the small bowel and caecum packed upwards from the pelvis. With the sigmoid colon retracted to the left, the right ureter is identified as it crosses the iliac vessels and an incision in the overlying peritoneum is carried downwards into the pelvis.

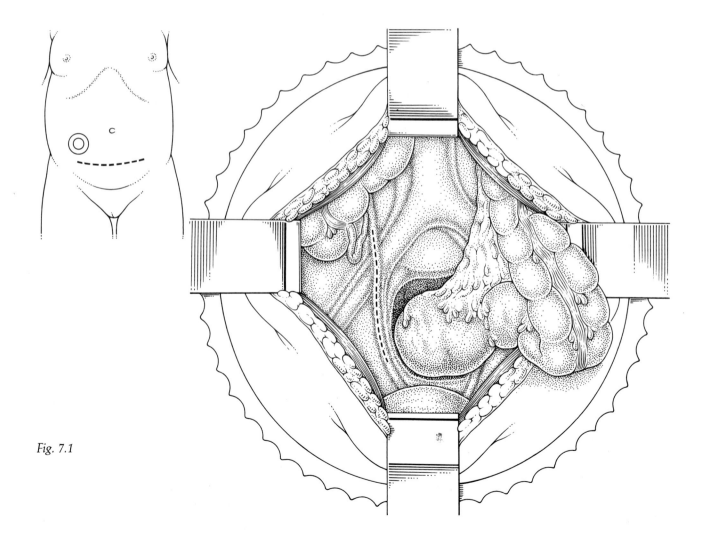

Fig. 7.1

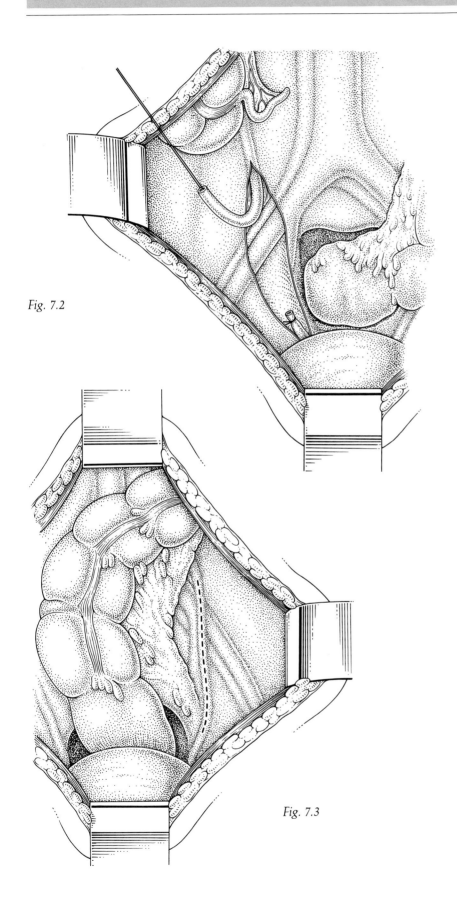

Fig. 7.2

Fig. 7.3

The pelvic ureter is mobilized along with its surrounding adventitia, ligated close to the bladder with an absorbable suture, and divided (Fig. 7.2).

The sigmoid colon is retracted to the right and the left ureter similarly identified and mobilized (Fig. 7.3).

Formation of an ileal conduit (Fig. 7.4)
The conduit need be based only on a single major vessel, usually the last intestinal branch of the superior mesenteric artery (although more proximal branches may be used if indicated), and this should be sited towards the proximal end of the conduit. The length of conduit should be minimal—no more than the distance between posterior abdominal wall and stoma site plus 3–5 cm extra to allow for construction of an everted stoma. After marking the extremities with tissue forceps, the appropriate vessels are ligated and divided. Proximally these comprise only the outer two arcades, while distally all arcades are divided and the mesentery incised well down towards its base. Intestinal clamps (not illustrated) are placed and the bowel divided at each end between them.

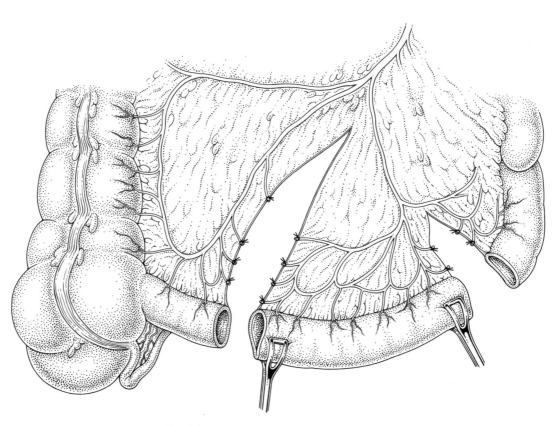

Fig. 7.4

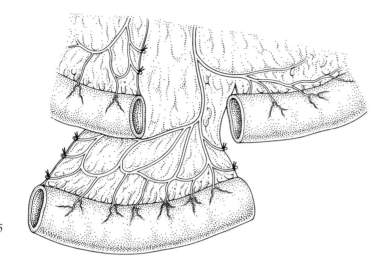

Fig. 7.5

The conduit is swung infero-medially on its mesentery before restoring intestinal continuity (Fig. 7.5).

In young children, intestinal continuity is restored with all-layer interrupted horizontal mattress sutures of 3/0 silk (Fig. 7.6).

In older children a conventional two-layer anastomosis is performed with a running all-layer 3/0 chromic catgut suture reinforced with interrupted 3/0 silk seromuscular sutures. The mesenteric defect is closed with further sutures (Fig. 7.7).

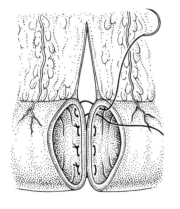

Fig. 7.6

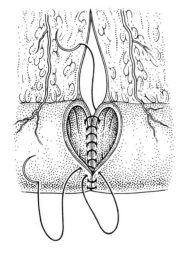

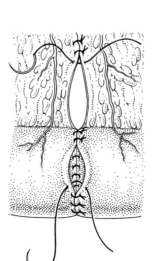

Fig. 7.7

A tunnel is developed beneath the retroperitoneum and sigmoid mesentery, commencing just above the pelvic brim and running slightly upwards from right to left. The left ureter is drawn through this tunnel (Fig. 7.8) and may be freed proximally on its lateral aspect for a few centimetres so that it describes a smooth curve towards the right.

Formation of a sigmoid conduit (Fig. 7.9)

The sigmoid loop is mobilized by dividing the peritoneum laterally at the base of its mesentery. The conduit can be based on a single sigmoid vessel but, because sigmoid colon tends to contract once isolated, its length should be slightly greater than for a corresponding ileal conduit. The extremities of the conduit are marked with tissue forceps, the marginal artery ligated and divided at each end and the mesentery incised toward its base. Bowel clamps (not illustrated) are placed and the colon is divided at either end between them. Before restoring intestinal continuity, the conduit may be swung medially or laterally on its mesentery; the former is usually more satisfactory. The colon is anastomosed by either of the methods described in Figures 7.6 and 7.7. If the conduit lies laterally, the right ureter is brought to the left in the reverse manner to that illustrated in Figure 7.8; if it lies medially, both ureters are brought retroperitoneally to an incision in the retroperitoneum placed medial to the sigmoid mesentery just above the pelvic brim.

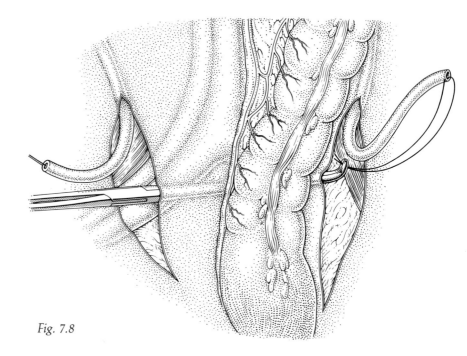

Fig. 7.8

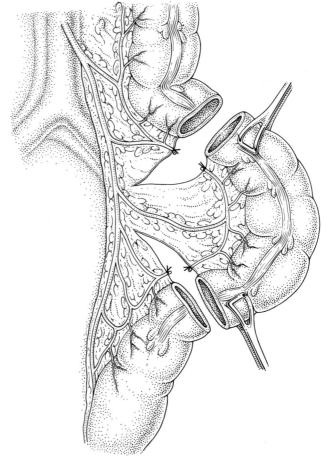

Fig. 7.9

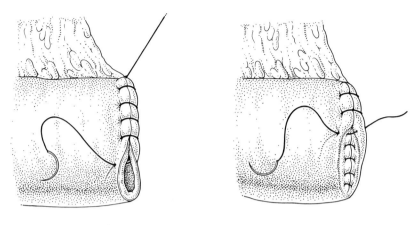

Fig. 7.10

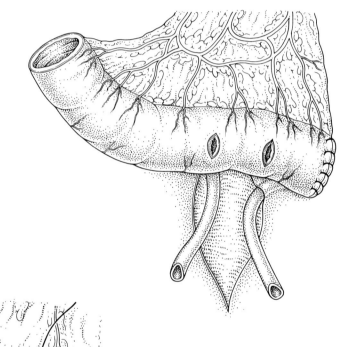

Fig. 7.11

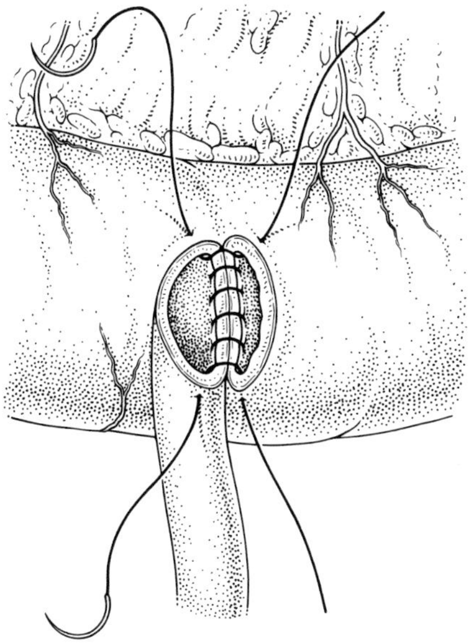

Refluxing ureterointestinal anastomoses

The Bricker (1950) and Wallace (1970) anastomoses are described. In the long term the results are similar but the Wallace method has given fewer short-term complications in the author's hands.

The Bricker technique (Fig. 7.10). The proximal end of the conduit is closed with a running all-layer 3/0 chromic catgut suture reinforced by interrupted 3/0 polyglycolic acid seromuscular sutures.

Both ureters are spatulated and corresponding full-thickness incisions are made in the conduit close to its anti-mesenteric border (Fig. 7.11).

One side of the anastomosis is completed with 3—4 all-layer 4/0 chromic catgut sutures with knots placed externally (Fig. 7.12). A transanastomotic splint (if used) is inserted at this stage.

Fig. 7.12

The opposite side of the anastomosis is similarly constructed (Fig. 7.13).

The second ureterointestinal anastomosis is completed and the proximal end of the conduit anchored to the retroperitoneal tissues with 4–5 absorbable sutures (Fig. 7.14).

The Wallace technique (Fig. 7.15). The ureters are brought together transversely side by side and their anterior aspects incised for a distance slightly greater than the diameter of the conduit.

The posterior uretero-ureteral anastomosis is formed with a running 3/0 or 4/0 chromic catgut suture (Fig. 7.16).

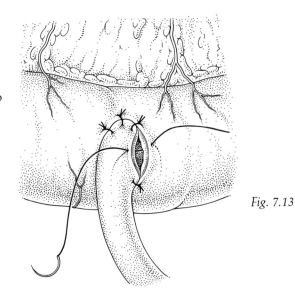

Fig. 7.13

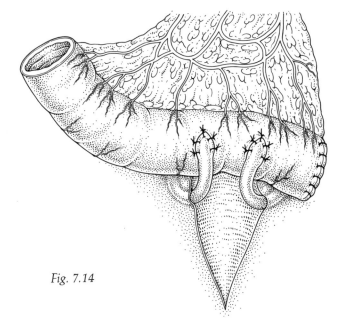

Fig. 7.14

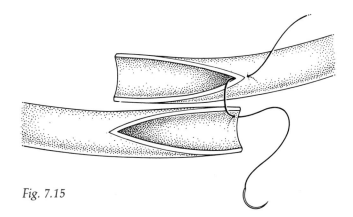

Fig. 7.15

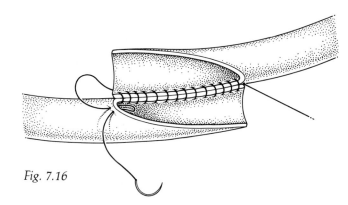

Fig. 7.16

The suture line is run anteriorly from either end until the aperture in the conjoined ureters corresponds to the diameter of the conduit (Fig. 7.17).

The proximal end of the conduit is anastomosed to the conjoined ureters with a running all-layer 3/0 chromic catgut suture (Fig. 7.18). Ureteric splints (if used) are placed before completing the interior aspect of the anastomosis. The incised retroperitoneum may be sutured around the base of the conduit so that the ureterointestinal anastomosis lies extraperitoneally.

Sometimes a better ureteric 'lie' is obtained if the ureters are brought together vertically rather than transversely (Fig. 7.19).

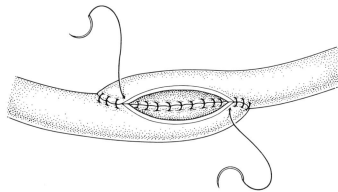

Fig. 7.17

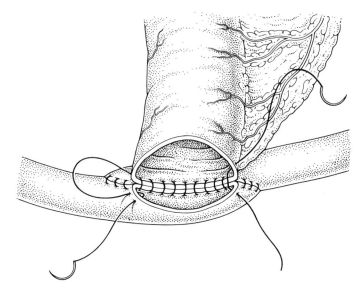

Fig. 7.18

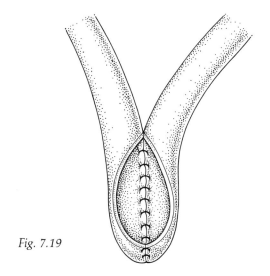

Fig. 7.19

Non-refluxing ureterointestinal anastomoses

Non-refluxing anastomoses are usually constructed with sigmoid colon although Mathisen buds may be made from ileum. Ureters dilated to a diameter of 1 cm or more will require tailoring for 4–6 cm by the method described in Chapter 5.

Leadbetter anastomosis (Leadbetter & Clarke 1954, Fig. 7.20). Traction sutures steady the conduit or the colon in continuity at the region of the anastomosis. A 4–5 cm incision along a taenia is deepened to the extramucosal plane.

The seromuscular layers are raised from the mucosa by blunt dissection for 1–1.5 cm on each side. Traction sutures aid this process. The ureter is spatulated and a corresponding incision is made vertically through the colonic mucosa (Fig. 7.21).

The anastomosis is commenced using 4/0 chromic catgut sutures (Fig. 7.22).

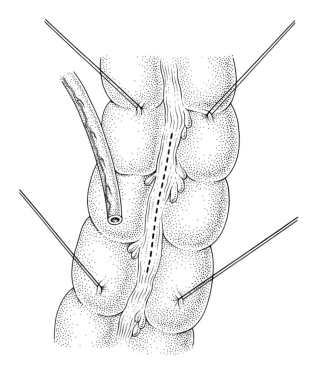

Fig. 7.20

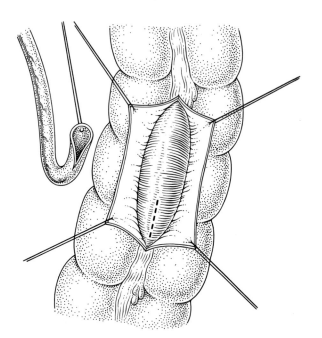

Fig. 7.21

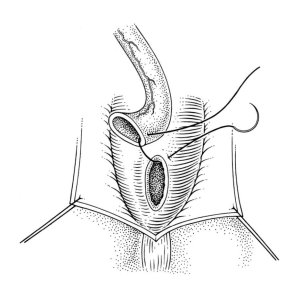

Fig. 7.22

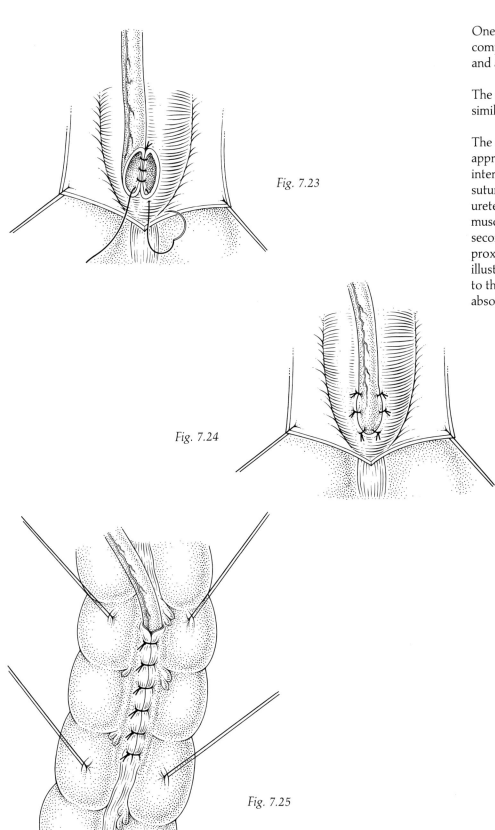

Fig. 7.23

Fig. 7.24

Fig. 7.25

One side of the anastomosis is completed with 3–4 sutures (Fig. 7.23), and a splint is passed at this stage.

The opposite side of the anastomosis is similarly constructed (Fig. 7.24).

The seromuscular flaps are approximated over the distal ureter with interrupted 4/0 polyglycolic acid sutures, taking care not to compress the ureter as it emerges from the sero-muscular tunnel (Fig. 7.25). After the second anastomosis is complete, the proximal end of a conduit is closed as illustrated in Figure 7.10 and anchored to the retroperitoneal tissues with 4–5 absorbable sutures.

The Mathisen bud technique (Mathisen 1953, Fig. 7.26). A full-thickness rectangular flap is cut in the conduit (or in the colon if ureterosigmoidostomy in continuity is being performed) some 2 cm in length and slightly greater than the ureteric circumference in width. The ureter is spatulated and sutured to the apex of the flap with a 4/0 chromic catgut suture which is held as a stay until completion of the bud.

Three further sutures wrap the apex of the flap around the ureter and the bud is completed by 3–4 more sutures which pick up all layers of the flap and the underlying ureteric adventitia (Fig. 7.27). A transanastomotic splint is placed at this stage.

The bud is inserted into the lumen of the bowel and the wall closed with all-layer interrupted 3/0 polyglycolic acid sutures which may be reinforced, if thought necessary, with a further layer of seromuscular sutures (Fig. 7.28). Care must be taken to avoid constricting the ureter as it emerges from the conduit. The second bud is constructed on the opposite side of the conduit at a slightly higher or slightly lower level. The proximal end of the conduit is closed (see Fig. 7.10) and anchored to the retroperitoneum.

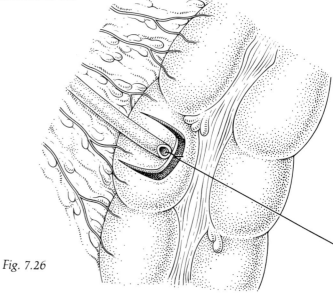

Fig. 7.26

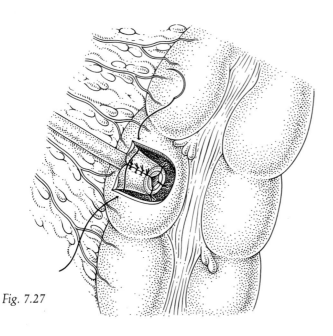

Fig. 7.27

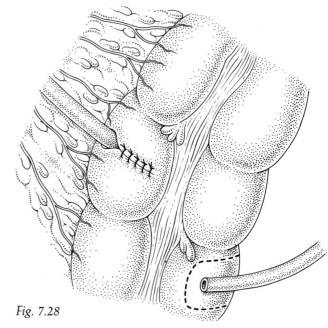

Fig. 7.28

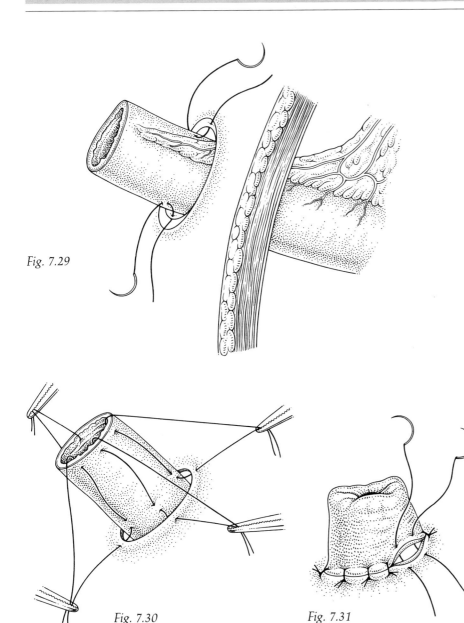

Fig. 7.29

Formation of a conduit stoma

Conduits may be brought extra- or transperitoneally; the latter is simpler and less prone to complications.

A circle of skin slightly greater than the diameter of the conduit is excised at the stoma site. Haemostats grasping peritoneum and rectus sheath on the upper margin of the wound are held so that deeper dissection passes vertically through the abdominal wall. Subcutaneous fat, muscle layers and peritoneum are incised in cruciate fashion and the conduit is grasped with tissue forceps and drawn through to the stoma site (Fig. 7.29). Four 3/0 or 2/0 chromic catgut sutures anchor the peritoneum to the seromuscular layers of the conduit.

Four 2/0 polyglycolic acid sutures are placed as shown in Figure 7.30, picking up skin, conduit serosa and all layers at the mouth of the conduit.

These sutures are tied to form an everted stoma projecting some 2–3 cm, and further sutures approximate skin to the outer wall of the eversion (Fig. 7.31).

Stomal stenosis is a common complication and the risk can be lessened if, rather than excising a circle of skin, flaps are incorporated around the stoma (Smith 1972, Fig. 7.32).

Fig. 7.30

Fig. 7.31

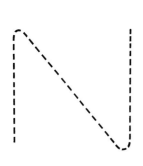
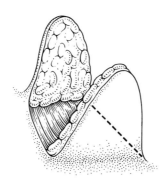
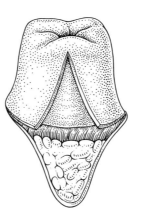
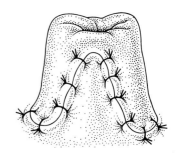

Fig. 7.32

Terminal ureterostomy (Fig. 7.33)
If there is disparity between the size of
the ureters, the larger is brought out as
the stoma and the smaller anastomosed
to it as a transuretero-ureterostomy (Fig.
7.33).

If both ureters are massively dilated,
they may be brought out together as a
double-barrelled stoma (Fig. 7.34).

The ureters are mobilized as illustrated
in Figures 7.1–7.3 and 7.8. Care must be
taken to preserve ureteric vasculature
and any kinks in the distal ureters
should be straightened by cautious
division of the flimsy adhesions which
unite adjacent portions of ureter. A 'V'
incision at the stoma site is deepened to
extraperitoneal level, from where a
tunnel is created by blunt dissection to
the retroperitoneum (Fig. 7.35). The
more dilated ureter is brought to the
surface through this tunnel and should
describe a smooth curve throughout.

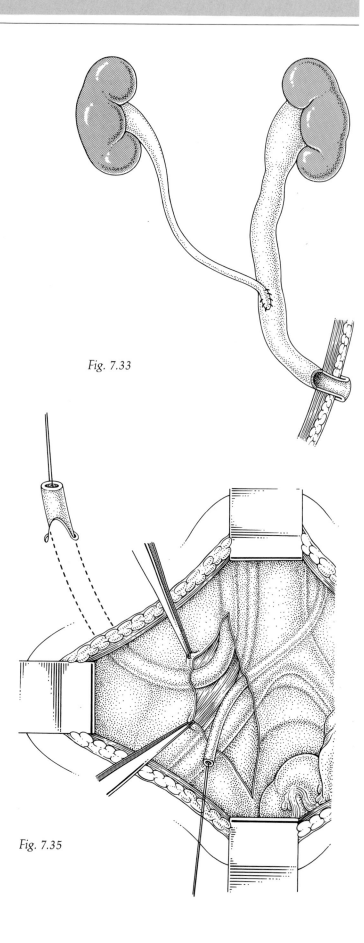

Fig. 7.33

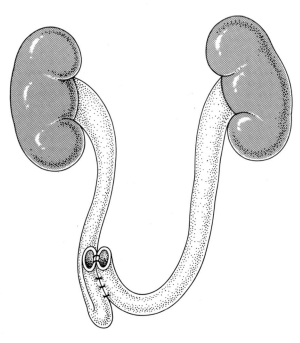

Fig. 7.34

Fig. 7.35

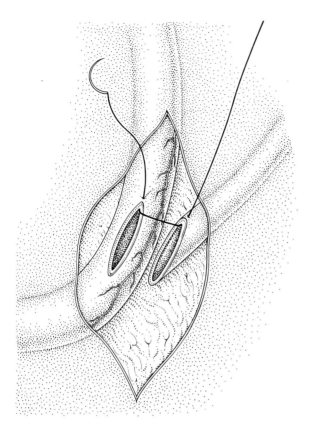

Fig. 7.36

The smaller ureter is spatulated and a corresponding incision made in the larger ureter away from major ureteric vessels (Fig. 7.36).

The posterior aspect of the transuretero-ureterostomy is constructed with all-layer 3/0 or 4/0 chromic catgut sutures (Fig. 7.37).

The anterior aspect of the anastomosis is completed and the retroperitoneum closed over it (Fig. 7.38).

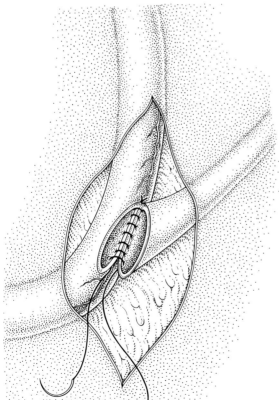

Fig. 7.37

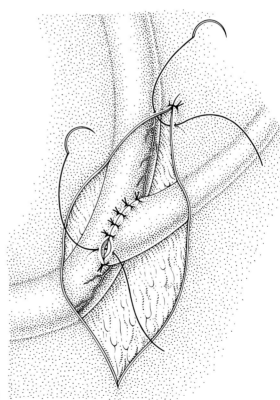

Fig. 7.38

If possible, an everted stoma is made, projecting some 1–1.5 cm, and the risk of stenosis is minimized if a 'V' skin flap is incorporated into the eversion (Fig. 7.39). The stoma is sutured to skin with 3/0 or 4/0 polyglycolic acid sutures.

Ureterosigmoidostomy in continuity
(Goodwin et al 1953, Fig. 7.40). The ureters are mobilized as illustrated in Figures 7.1–7.3. The lower sigmoid colon is opened anteriorly for some 8 cm along a taenia coli. Traction sutures in the posterior sigmoid mucosa mark the sites of entry of the ureters and the distal limits of the proposed submucosal tunnels. Through an incision in the posterior wall of the sigmoid colon, a haemostat is advanced retroperitoneally to grasp a traction suture on the ureter.

The ureter is drawn into the colon and advanced distally in a 3–4 cm submucosal tunnel (Fig. 7.41).

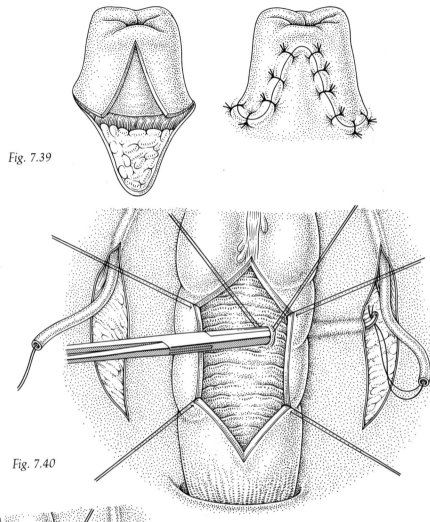

Fig. 7.39

Fig. 7.40

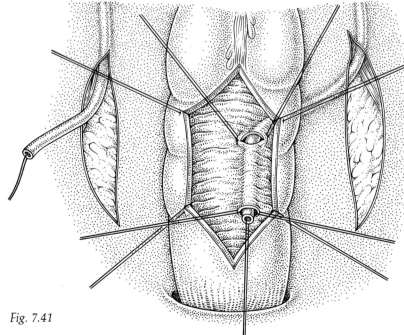

Fig. 7.41

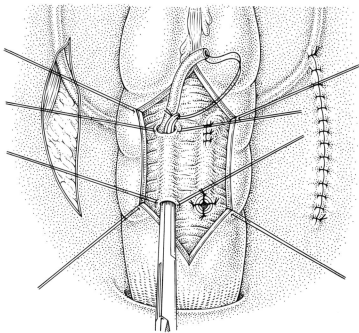

Fig. 7.42

The ureter is spatulated and anastomosed to colonic mucosa with 4/0 chromic catgut sutures (Fig. 7.42). Similar sutures close the proximal incision in the colonic mucosa. The colon is closed with a running 2/0 or 3/0 chromic catgut suture, reinforced with interrupted 3/0 silk seromuscular stitches.

The ureters may also be anastomosed for ureterosigmoidostomy by the Leadbetter or Mathisen methods.

Drainage after urinary diversion
Transanastomotic ureteric drainage to the exterior is advisable with ureterosigmoidostomy in continuity, with non-refluxing conduit anastomoses and if the ureters have been tailored. 4–8F umbilical catheters or infant feeding tubes may be used and should be anchored at the anastomosis with a chromic catgut suture and brought through the stoma or the anus. Alternatively, pig-tailed stents may be employed. A rectal tube should be inserted after ureterosigmoidostomy. Ureteric splints are optional after other forms of diversion but, if not used, the anastomoses must be externally drained intra- or extraperitoneally as appropriate.

REFERENCES

Althausen A F, Hagen-Cook K, Hendren W H 1978 Non-refluxing colon conduit: experience with 70 cases. Journal of Urology 120: 35–39

Bricker E M 1950 Bladder substitution after pelvic exenteration. Surgical Clinics of North America 30: 1511–1521

Goodwin W E, Harris A P, Kaufmann J J, Beal J M 1953 Open, transcolonic ureterointestinal anastomosis; new approach. Surgery, Gynecology and Obstetrics 97: 295–300

Leadbetter W F, Clarke B G 1954 Five years experience with uretero-enterostomy by the 'combined' technique. Journal of Urology 73: 67–82

Mathisen W 1953 A new method for ureterointestinal anastomosis. Surgery, Gynecology and Obstetrics 96: 255–258

Middleton A W, Hendren W H 1976 Ileal conduits at the Massachusetts General Hospital from 1955 to 1970. Journal of Urology 115: 591–595

Smith E D 1972 Follow-up studies of 150 ileal conduits in children. Journal of Pediatric Surgery 7: 1–10

Stewart M 1986 Urinary diversion and bowel cancer. Annals of the Royal College of Surgeons of England 68: 98–102

Wallace D M 1970 Uretero-ileostomy. British Journal of Urology 42: 529–534

Chapter 8

Undiversion—indications and patient assessment

Timothy P. Stephenson

Introduction

There is now a wealth of literature on undiversion stretching back 15 years (Hendren 1973). It remains a fascinating area of reconstructive surgery because methods of assessment, techniques of augmentation and substitution of the bladder, the use of an increasingly reliable sphincter prosthesis and wide acceptance of self-intermittent catheterization have made it possible to undivert safely almost all patients with a surface diversion. It must be said also that many of the techniques described a decade or more ago by Hendren (1974, 1976) have stood the test of time, and there is no finer series than his recent report of 150 patients undiverted since 1969 (Hendren 1987).

In most centres involved in reconstructive surgery, undiversion has become comparatively rare because most of the pool of suitable patients have been reconstructed and all those patients who now present themselves who would previously have been diverted are reconstructed as the primary procedure, though we still have a handful every year. Clearly the same techniques will apply to both groups.

PATIENT SELECTION FOR UNDIVERSION

The great majority of patients assessed for undiversion in our own unit are referred initially with medical problems. Most have myelomeningoceles, which has a high prevalence in Wales for reasons unknown, and are cared for by a dedicated and experienced team who involve us when necessary. Most commonly this results from upper tract deterioration due to some or all of the complications of a long-term diversion—stomal stenosis, stasis in the loop, chronic infection, stones and reflux. In such cases surgery is mandatory, though whether undiversion or conversion to a continent diversion is the procedure of choice depends on the ambulatory status, body configuration and the intelligence and motivation of the patient.

At the other end of the spectrum is the non-ambulatory child with normal upper tracts, a good stoma, without appliance problems or recurrent infections, and with limited intelligence in whom undiversion is never considered. However, because of the 'family' nature of the spina bifida environment, parents occasionally request undiversion for their child because of knowledge of a successful result in another child. Very careful counselling of such parents is required.

Between these two ends of the spectrum are a number of patients who have less serious problems such as occasional infections, minor appliance problems and poor psychological adjustment to their stoma, especially in teenagers on the threshold of sexual activity. Very careful psychosocial assessment is required in the latter, particularly in relation to their expectations, and to underline, especially in the more difficult cases, that failure is a possibility after a lot of major surgery has been undertaken. We remain reluctant to

undivert for purely social reasons except in the non-neuropath where the reconstruction is (almost) certain to be straightforward. There is also a small group of patients diverted as babies for whom diversion is normality and who refuse undiversion despite significant medical indications. It is important to recognize that some of the spina bifida group seem, on superficial discussion, more intelligent and motivated than they really are, and undiversion in some of these may result in problems if intermittent catheterization or an artificial sphincter is required. In such patients who have relative rather than absolute indications for reconstruction, apart from a careful assessment of the patient himself, it is also fundamental to develop a good relationship with the parent(s) who are often protective and suspicious of surgery and surgeons. No decision is taken about reconstruction in these patients until both supratentorial and complete anatomical and functional assessment of the lower urinary tract has been completed.

Although the great majority of our undiversions are in patients with neuropathy (35 of 43), there is a handful of benign and malignant cases and, if there is an absolute indication for surgery (i.e. deteriorating upper tracts), even radical cystectomy and partial urethrectomy do not preclude undiversion (see below).

ANATOMICAL AND FUNCTIONAL ASSESSMENT OF PATIENTS BEFORE UNDIVERSION

The aims of undiversion have been stated many times but bear repeating:

1. Preservation or improvement of the upper tracts;
2. Adequate bladder capacity;
3. Maintenance of low detrusor pressure during bladder filling;
4. Reflux prevention;
5. Achievement of complete, efficient voiding;
6. Maintenance or establishment of continence.

Renal function
Renography should be performed and serum creatinine estimated to determine renal function. There is a cut-off point at about a creatinine of 250–300 mg% at which it becomes more difficult to stabilize renal function, partly because such patients always have adynamic ureters, partly because if bowel is used in the reconstruction some resorption occurs, and partly in some instances intrinsic renal disease and hypertension perpetuate renal impairment. Nevertheless, no patient in advanced renal failure is rejected for undiversion if young since it is very much better to transplant into a satisfactory reconstruction than into a diversion which may have contributed to the renal failure in the first place (see below).

Ureteric function and anatomy
The lengths of the proximal ureters and distal ureteric stumps should be determined by excretory urography, videocystography and, if necessary, retrograde ureterograms. The most important study in those with impaired renal function may be fluoroscopy of the ureters during excretory urography to assess the peristaltic activity of the ureters (or absence thereof), for this is fundamental in the planning of the reconstruction. The presence of reflux into the distal ureteric stumps is usually unimportant as it most often resolves after reconstruction.

Bladder anatomy and function
The defunctionalized bladder is always small and contracted but usually thin-walled and supple, even in the neuropath, and a period of hydrostatic cycling will often produce a remarkable increase in bladder capacity in a fairly short time. Until the advent of the 'clam'

(see Chapter 9) procedure it was our policy with the neuropath to excise routinely all but the trigone and perform a substitution cystoplasty. Currently it is our policy to persist with bladder cycling until no further increase in volume can be achieved and, if a capacity of at least 150 ml can be obtained, the clam procedure is usually feasible, since these bladders are rarely fibrotic and sacculated. Serial flow rates and residual urine measurements via a suprapubic catheter may be more helpful than urodynamics in the non-neuropath both in terms of assessment of voiding efficiency and continence.

In the neuropath a more detailed evaluation is required as regards bladder-filling pressures, voiding pressures and the visual assessment of the sphincter mechanism during voiding or attempted voiding.

Urethral anatomy and function
Techniques such as the electromyogram and dynamic and static pressure profiles have been abandoned and the clinical decisions about treatment of the outflow are based on serial cycling and subsequent videocystometry.

Cysto-urethroscopy is an essential part of the assessment but in the neuropath is postponed until the decision as to whether self-intermittent catheterization (SIC) or an artificial sphincter is going to be the method of achieving voiding. If the former is the method of choice, the child is taught the technique of SIC at this stage. A routine cysto-urethroscopy is performed, but if SIC proved difficult or psychologically unacceptable (as is quite common in the UK), radical sphincterotomy is performed at the time of the endoscopy in preparation for re-construction with an artificial sphincter at a later date. Occasionally it is possible to achieve adequate voiding and maintain continence by selective sphincterotomy, which may need repeating at least once on the premise

that it is better to repeat the procedure and maintain continence than to divide too much sphincter initially and lose continence.

If radical sphincterotomy has been performed it is essential to repeat video-cystometry before definitive re-construction. This is mainly to ensure that sphincterotomy is complete, for there is no more dangerous hazard to a reconstruction than having to carry out a further sphincterotomy once a sphincter cuff is in place because of the risk of exposing the cuff.

TECHNIQUES OF UNDIVERSION

Most surgeons involved in the re-construction of the lower urinary tract have changed their techniques over the past few years and will no doubt continue to do so, though it is difficult to see radical alterations until and unless a satisfactory artificial bladder is produced. The following discussion represents our personal approach to the various problems presented by the need for undiversion, though everyone would now agree that some form of de-tubularization is virtually always required.

Patients with anatomically and functionally normal lower urinary tract of adequate capacity
In this small group, continuity can be restored by a small variety of straight-forward procedures—psoas hitch plus uretero-ureterostomy or use of part of the loop itself if the gap is too great, or a new segment of small bowel if necessary. Like most reconstructions there is a period between 6 weeks and 3 months when urography may show some increase in upper tract distension, which settles with time.

Patients with neuropathy and adequate cycled bladder capacity ($> 150 \text{ cm}^3$)
Most of these bladders are fairly thin-walled and compliant. It is the continued presence of urine flow in an obstructed lower urinary tract that creates the thick-walled, sacculated fibrotic bladder that comes to substitution cystoplasty.

The bladder is split in the sagittal plane as for any clam and the posterior is half-hitched to the psoas. If the patient has an ileal loop, ideally the proximal part of the loop carrying the ureters is tapered and laid into the posterior wall of the bladder (Hendren 1976). If the diversion was by cutaneous ureterostomy and the ureters are acontractile, a new segment of ileum is used in similar fashion and, likewise, if a colon loop has been used this is abandoned and again replaced with tapered ileum.

If the ureters are peristaltic, of reasonable calibre and will reach the posterior wall, a tunnelled reimplant is the procedure of choice.

A large segment of ileum is isolated and a routine clam performed across the tapered ileum or ureter. If an artificial sphincter is being implanted the bladder neck is dissected before the clam is sewn into place, and after the anastomoses are completed the abdomen is flushed with the antibiotic solution, Taurodoline, and gloves and suitable drapes changed before the sphincter components are implanted. This procedure is satisfactory whatever the state of the upper tracts, even with aperistaltic ureters, for we have never had a 'Hendren' reimplant cause obstruction, and this is the procedure of choice with poor quality or short ureters.

Patients with non-distensible or very thick-walled sacculated bladders
Occasionally, previously 'normal' bladders simply will not significantly increase in size. There is a small group

of patients diverted for interstitial cystitis or chronic inflammation of unknown cause (and usually with reflux and hydronephrosis) who have small, fibrotic, inflamed bladders; and the exstrophy bladders, though usually supple, are tiny and often used to form the neo-urethra. Finally, the thickened, sacculated, neuropathic bladder is unsuitable for the clam, but is rare in the undiversion group though common in the primary reconstruction situation. In these, a large detubularized segment of caecum is used (see Chapter 9). If the ureters are normal they can be nippled into the ileal tail or tunnelled into the caecum, but if they are aperistaltic, they are either 'trouser-legged' into the ileal tail with or without reinforcement of the ileo-caecal valve or, if the loop is suitable, it can itself be nippled into the caecum, stapled and sutured to an appropriate denuded area. If a sphincter is being implanted, the same precautions described above apply.

Patients who have had a cystectomy
In our hands undiversion in this group is limited to those who have an absolute indication for surgery, such as deteriorating renal function, and in whom continent diversion is inappropriate or refused. In the male, provided there is some urethra left, it is usually possible to bridge the gap between a detubularized caeco-cystoplasty and even the bulbar urethra with small bowel, and low-pressure sphincters around the bowel appear safe. In women, the situation is more difficult, but again a low-pressure sphincter may be used around ileum or caecum, and there are non-prosthetic techniques available to create continence and SIC (Mundy 1988).

Undiversion and transplantation
Fifteen per cent of our overall experience in undiversion has involved subsequent planned transplantation, and there are a small number of undiversions

with poor renal function who may come to transplantation in the future. All but two of the undiversion/transplantation group have been neuropaths and have had substitution cystoplasties (though they would now be 'clammed' if appropriate). Although two have artificial sphincters, SIC is preferable because of the potentially greater risk of infection in the immunosuppressed patient. In only one, selective sphincterotomy achieved balanced voiding. Careful planning and cooperation between urologist, transplant surgeon, nephrologist, anaesthetist and intensivist are required. If the reconstruction is complex, it is desirable for the transplant surgeon to see the anatomy before wound closure in order to plan the siting of the transplant and the ureteric implantation, and it is sometimes useful for the urologist to assist with the ureteric insertion. It is desirable to implant the donor kidney as soon as the reconstruction is healed so that the material or substituted bladder remains 'dry' for as short a time as possible, especially if a mucus-producing bowel segment has been used. Thus a living related donor is preferable to facilitate this sequence.

Where a caecocystoplasty has been used, the proximal loop plus the stump of one ureter may be anastomosed to the ileal tail and a subsequent ureteroureterostomy performed at the time of transplantation; this is still a useful technique when substitution is indicated. Omental wrapping is considered mandatory because of the poor healing properties in renal failure. The one death in our series resulted from breakdown of the ileo-colic anastomosis. In another patient in whom most of the omentum had been removed, a cutaneous fistula developed at the vesico-colic anastomosis which was closed with a strip of the remaining omentum swung on the right gastro-epiploic vessels.

If a donor kidney is not available, the suprapubic catheter is left in situ and the natural bladder cycled to maintain capacity, or the substitution bladder is irrigated daily to prevent mucus accumulation. Voiding difficulties post transplant should not be a problem since balanced voiding must be established before transplantation (underlined by the fact that we are often asked to evaluate transplant patients who *do* have voiding problems after transplantation).

This transplant group has proved to be the most challenging and rewarding in the undiversion spectrum because of good results achieved in most patients and the interest of working with a multidisciplinary group. Even in patients clearly destined for end-stage renal failure, it is better to undivert early since healing is better and the problems of the 'dry' bladder are avoided.

CONCLUSIONS

Improved understanding of the lower urinary tract and of the way isolated bowel segments will behave, a reasonably reliable artificial sphincter and better pharmacological agents, plus an acceptance even in the UK of self-intermittent catheterization have made most undiversions fairly straight-forward. Nevertheless, meticulous care is needed in assessment, surgery and postoperative care.

Long-term follow-up is essential, partly because of the lessons taught by supravesical diversion and partly because of the tiny but possible risk of tumour formation (Stone et al 1987). However, it does seem that undiversion and primary reconstruction are going to prove safer in terms of avoiding such upper tract problems as stones, infections and renal deterioration than diversion has been, even apart from its social advantages.

REFERENCES

Hendren W H 1973 Reconstruction of previously diverted urinary tracts in children. Journal of Pediatric Surgery 8: 135

Hendren W H 1974 Urinary tract refunctionalisation after prior diversion in children. Annals of Surgery 180: 494

Hendren W H 1976 Urinary diversion and undiversion in children. Surgical Clinics of North America 56: 425

Hendren W H 1987 Techniques for urinary undiversion. In: Bladder reconstruction and continent urinary diversion. Year Book Medical Publishers, Chicago, p 101

Mundy A R 1988 A technique for total substitution of the lower urinary tract without the use of a prosthesis. British Journal of Urology 42: 334–338

Stone A R, Davies N, Stephenson T P 1987 Carcinoma associated with augmentation cystoplasty. British Journal of Urology 60: 236–238

Chapter 9

Augmentation and substitution cystoplasty

A. R. Mundy

Introduction

There are two types of cystoplasty: augmentation cystoplasty in which the bladder is enlarged, and substitution cystoplasty in which it is replaced. They are both uncommon procedures outside specializing units and are usually only used as a last resort for an otherwise intractable lower urinary tract problem for which the only alternative is some form of urinary diversion. The commonest indication in paediatric practice for both procedures is detrusor dysfunction due to spina bifida and the commonest complication after both is voiding imbalance, often giving exactly the same symptoms as the patient had beforehand. For this reason it is easy to ascribe a poor result to refractory disease rather than to inadequate surgery but it is inadequate surgery due to failure to understand the principles of cystoplasty that is responsible for most poor results.

INDICATIONS

The indications for both procedures are similar, the main difference being one of degree. The usual indications are detrusor dysfunction, the small contracted bladder and, for substitution cystoplasty, selected cases of lower urinary tract malignancy.

Detrusor dysfunction

There are three main types of detrusor dysfunction for which cystoplasty may be appropriate: poor bladder compliance, refractory detrusor instability and detrusor hyperreflexia.

Poor compliance may be seen on urodynamic testing in children with small capacity bladders whatever the cause, in some children with detrusor instability as a consequence of outflow obstruction (past or present), particularly in relation to posterior urethral valves, and in children with neuropathic dysfunction (Mundy 1985a).

Refractory detrusor instability and detrusor hyperreflexia are here taken to mean the occurrence of involuntary detrusor contractions on urodynamic testing that have not responded to the full range of conservative treatment modalities (Mundy 1985b, c). Instability is the term used in the absence of an overt neuropathy; hyperreflexia is used when the child has an overt neuropathy to account for the vesico-urethral dysfunction.

Augmentation cystoplasty is appropriate for patients with poor bladder compliance in the absence of neuropathy (Mundy & Stephenson 1985), for refractory detrusor instability (Mundy 1985b, c, Mundy & Stephenson 1985) and for minor degrees of neuropathic dysfunction (poor compliance or detrusor hyper-

reflexia or both), usually when the thickness of the bladder wall is relatively normal.

Substitution cystoplasty is indicated when poor compliance is associated with gross thickening of the bladder wall and in severe degrees of neuropathic dysfunction (Stephenson & Mundy 1985).

In children without neuropathic dysfunction, age is obviously an important factor when considering surgical intervention and common sense dictates that cystoplasty should only be considered in teenagers with intractable symptoms who are past the age when a natural spontaneous resolution of their symptoms could be expected.

The commonest 'non-neuropathic' group is that of children with a bladder dysfunction that looks 'neuropathic' on investigation of the lower urinary tract but with no clinical evidence of an overt neuropathy, particularly when the lower tract abnormality appears to be causing upper tract complications.

The small contracted bladder

In paediatric practice this is usually related to detrusor dysfunction, but one occasionally sees children with small contracted bladders for no apparent reason or following some previous surgical misadventure.

Other indications

These include conditions such as previous and adequately treated lower urinary tract malignancy, usually rhabdomyosarcoma, bladder exstrophy when there is insufficient bladder tissue for a simple closure, and other situations that have left the bladder in a similar state.

In practice, by far the largest group of children to be considered for cystoplasty are those with congenital cord lesions, particularly spina bifida, and here it is important to remember that, in addition to the bladder dysfunction, there is almost invariably a degree of sphincter dysfunction that will also need attention. The decision as to which type of cystoplasty should be performed depends on the bladder capacity, the thickness of the bladder wall and the presence or absence of vesico-ureteric junction (VUJ) obstruction as a consequence of the bladder wall abnormality. Those children with a reasonable bladder capacity, a relatively normal bladder wall thickness and no upper tract abnormalities (the vast majority) will be treated by augmentation cystoplasty, and those with small, thick-walled bladders and VUJ obstruction will require substitution.

ASSESSMENT WITH A VIEW TO CYSTOPLASTY

The minimum requirements are an intravenous urogram (IVU), a video-urodynamic study (VUD) and a cysto-urethroscopy. The VUD provides the urodynamic diagnosis and an assessment of its severity, and the IVU shows whether there are secondary upper tract changes. If there are, and these are not due to reflux (which will be shown on the VUD), then a Tc-99mDTPA renal scan will show whether or not there is obstruction, and a repeat scan after a week or so of indwelling catheterization will show whether this is due to outflow obstruction, in which case the upper tract changes will resolve with catheterization, or to obstruction of the intramural ureters as they pass through a thickened or fibrotic bladder wall, in which case the upper tract obstruction will persist.

Cystourethroscopy allows the measurement of bladder capacity, the exclusion or need for treatment of outflow obstruction and the further assessment of trabeculation and sacculation (or any other intravesical pathology) (Mundy & Stephenson 1984a, Mundy 1985b), the severity of which may sway the surgeon towards substitution rather than augmentation cystoplasty.

PROBLEMS ASSOCIATED WITH CYSTOPLASTY

Apart from the usual complications of any major operation, there are three particular problems associated with cystoplasty which must be anticipated (Turner-Warwick 1976). The first two are voiding imbalance and 'diverticulization' of the cystoplasty segment. The choice of procedure, operative technique and further management are all influenced by these two factors. The third is due to the presence of an intestinal segment within the urinary tract and this is discussed at the end of the chapter.

Voiding imbalance
This is almost universal after either type of cystoplasty if bladder neck competence is unimpaired. (It is less common in girls than in boys because bladder neck incompetence is a common incidental abnormality in girls even in the absence of neuropathy. In neuropathy, bladder neck incompetence is very common.) For this reason it is advisable to perform a bladder neck incision routinely before, or at the time of, cystoplasty in a child with a competent bladder neck on VUD unless it is decided that the child is to use clean intermittent self-catheterization post-operatively and that no attempt is to be made to establish spontaneous voiding. Any residual voiding imbalance after the cystoplasty in either sex can be managed either by sphincter rebalancing

(Turner-Warwick 1976) or by clean intermittent self-catheterization (CISC) (Stephenson & Mundy 1985) or, in selected cases (mainly in neuropathic dysfunction when sphincteric obstruction can be difficult to manage otherwise), by sphincter ablation and implantation of an artificial urinary sphincter (AUS) (Mundy & Stephenson 1984b, Stephenson & Mundy 1985).

In children with urodynamically proven sphincter dysfunction, the decision as to which of three options is to be chosen should be made before undertaking the cystoplasty, as some children will be suitable for either selective sphincterotomy or sphincter ablation and implantation of an AUS at the time of their cystoplasty and because children to be managed by CISC should be proficient before their cystoplasty to avoid the problems of finding out that they cannot or will not do it afterwards when it is too late.

As a general rule the best option for the management of voiding imbalance after a cystoplasty is CISC. Bladder neck incision, sphincter rebalancing and sphincter ablation should be reserved for those instances where CISC is positively contraindicated.

Diverticulization of the cystoplasty segment
This tends to occur after both types of cystoplasty unless steps are taken to prevent it. In both instances it is usually due to contraction of the suture line by which the cystoplasty segment is sewn in place such that an 'hour glass' deformity develops. As described below, this is usually overcome by an almost complete bisection of the bladder before inlaying the cystoplasty segment in the augmentation procedure (Mundy & Stephenson 1985) and by making sure not to leave any more of the bladder than the trigone and bladder neck in substitution cystoplasty (Turner-Warwick 1976, Mundy 1986).

PREOPERATIVE PREPARATION

Patients for either procedure are admitted to hospital 4 days before operation. The preoperative regimen is the same for both procedures and consists of a mechanical and anti-microbial bowel preparation.

Day 4 preoperatively
Low residue diet
Oral magnesium sulphate 5–10 ml t.d.s.

Day 3 preoperatively
As for day 4

Day 2 preoperatively
As for day 4 *plus*
Morning and evening enema
Metronidazole 200–400 mg t.d.s.

Preoperative day
Fluids only
Magnesium sulphate 5–10 ml t.d.s.
Neomycin 1 g t.d.s.
Metronidazole 200–400 mg t.d.s.
Morning and evening enema

Day of operation
Parenteral gentamycin and metronidazole with the premedication and for 3–5 days after operation.

Sometimes, particularly in children with impaired renal function, there is a tendency to dehydration on the last day of preparation, and intravenous hydration will be necessary to prevent this.

AUGMENTATION CYSTOPLASTY

The technique described here is the one that the author uses routinely and almost exclusively using ileum (Bramble 1982, Mundy 1985b, c, Mundy & Stephenson 1985). In some situations it may seem easier to use the colon, particularly the sigmoid colon, to get a patch down into the pelvis on a vascular pedicle, but colonic anastomoses are far more prone to complications than ileal anastomoses and, coupled with the possible risk of a carcinoma developing in the colon when it is in contact with urine in the long term (Leadbetter et al 1979, Nurse & Mundy 1989a), this makes an ileocystoplasty preferable.

Incision

A midline lower abdominal, Pfannenstiel or suprapubic 'V' incision (Turner-Warwick et al 1974) may be used but the author prefers a Cherney incision (Cherney 1941) as this provides wide and easy access to the pelvis.

A curved skin incision (indicated by the dotted line in Fig. 9.1), as in the Pfannenstiel approach, is deepened down to the rectus sheath which is then incised similarly to expose the pyramidalis muscles and the underlying recti. The pyramidales are then reflected off the recti, with the rectus sheath, down to the anterior aspect of the pubis, exposing the rectus tendons as they insert into the pubis. The rectus tendons are then divided leaving just enough inferiorly for later closure, and the lateral fascial attachments of the recti to the deep aspect of the inguinal ligaments are then divided to allow the recti to be lifted up (Fig. 9.2). A ring retractor can then be placed to hold the incision open.

The retropubic space is widely opened to expose the pelvic floor all the way around the front and both lateral aspects of the bladder.

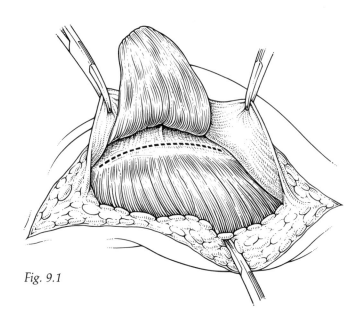

Fig. 9.1

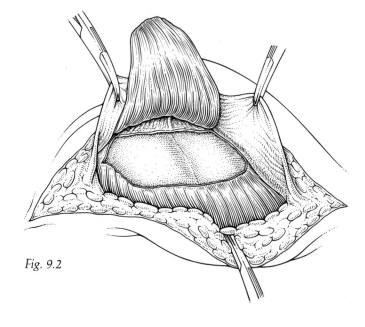

Fig. 9.2

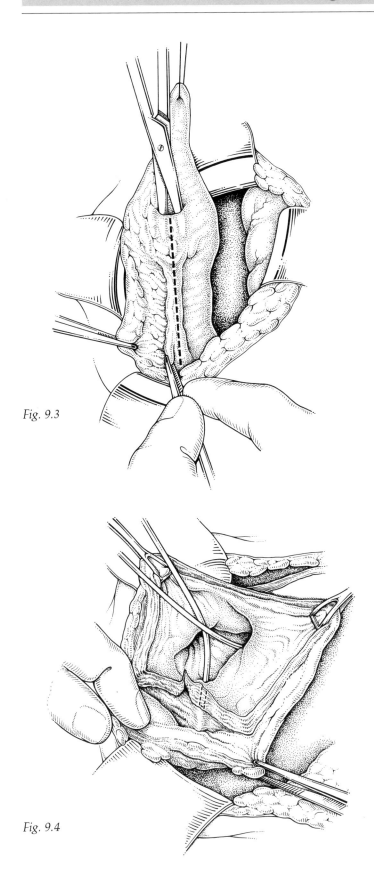

Fig. 9.3

Fig. 9.4

The urachus is then defined as it leaves the dome of the bladder and ligated and divided. The peritoneum just deep to this point is then opened to expose the dome of the bladder with its peritoneal covering.

Traction on the ligature that secures the urachus at the dome of the bladder and blunt dissection on either side will open up the plane of cleavage between the fascia on the lateral aspect of the bladder wall (anterior to the dotted line in Fig. 9.3) and the fascia and overlying peritoneum on the dome of the bladder (posterior to the dotted line in Fig. 9.3), where these two fascial layers join to run together as a single sheet to the brim of the pelvis along the line of the iliac vessels. Development of this plane of cleavage down along the lateral margin of the bladder to the ureter and superior vesical pedicle on each side exposes the maximal circumference of the bladder and allows the large veins that sometimes run in the fascia on the lateral bladder wall to be secured without much bleeding.

When the maximal circumference of the bladder has been exposed in this way, the bladder wall can be incised around its maximal circumference from a point 2 cm or so in front of the ureteric orifice and about 1 cm from the bladder neck on one side to a similar point on the other side. At this stage there should be a catheter in each ureter. This is most easily achieved by starting at the dome and working down on one side at a time (Fig. 9.4) using a diathermy point.

In this way the bladder is completely bisected except for a bridge of about 1 cm on either side of the bladder neck region (Fig. 9.5). In the figure, the circumference of the bisected bladder is being measured with a length of tubing (reproduced from Mundy & Stephenson 1985).

The cut edge of the bladder is then measured (which should be the same on both sides except that the bladder wall tends to contract down during the course of the procedure) and haemostasis is secured, particularly at the two ends of the incision in the bladder wall where a few significant vessels are likely to be encountered.

The next stage is to define and isolate a section of ileum on its vascular pedicle (Fig. 9.6). A convenient section of terminal ileum is selected that will drop down easily into the pelvis. It must be equal in length to the measured maximal circumference of the bladder and have a well-defined vascular arcade supplying it.

The ileum on either side is reconstituted in the usual way.

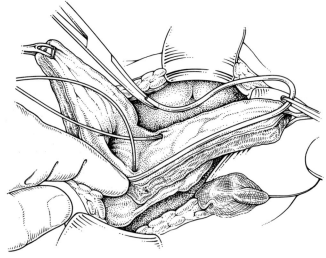

Fig. 9.5

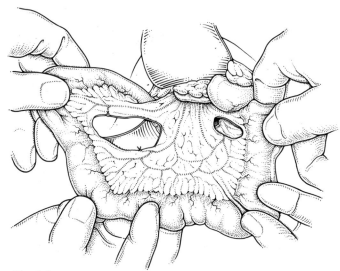

Fig. 9.6

Sometimes, although the mid-section of the ileal segment will reach easily to the bisected bladder, the natural upward curve of the two ends of the segment prevents them from reaching down to the two ends of the bladder bisection without tension. In this situation the mesenteric vessels in the proximal arcades at each side of the isolated segment must be ligated and divided in such a way as to allow the two ends of the ileum to drop down sufficiently. The ileal segment is then opened on its anti-mesenteric aspect to produce a patch (Fig. 9.7) and the two ends of this patch are triangulated.

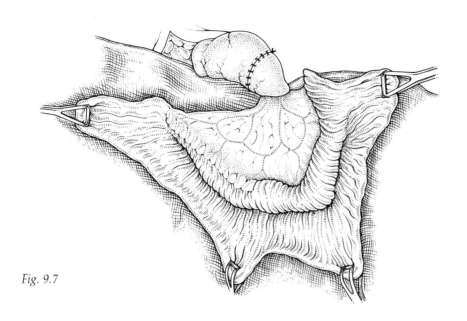

Fig. 9.7

The ileal patch is now inset into the bisected bladder and sewn in place. There is a tendency for the margins of the bladder to contract during the course of the procedure, producing an overlap between the ileal edge and the bladder edge during the anastomosis of the patch. To prevent this overlap from developing, each suture line is halved and then quartered with stay sutures and each quarter is then sewn up individually. The posterior suture line is dealt with first, from inside the bladder, using a continuous 2/0 or 3/0 vicryl stitch picking up the full thickness of the bladder and ileal walls, starting at the apex of the bladder incision in front of the ureter and working up on each side to the dome, locking to each of the 'quartering' stay stitches in turn as they are encountered. Figure 9.8 shows stay stitches at each end of the bladder (A), at the halfway mark (B) and halfway between on each side (C); the second quarter of the left side of the posterior suture line is nearing completion

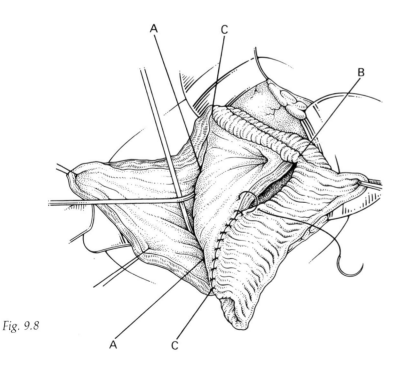

Fig. 9.8

When the posterior half of the anastomosis has been completed (Fig. 9.9, reproduced from Mundy & Stephenson 1985) the ileal patch is flipped over and the procedure is repeated, this time from outside the bladder, to sew the anterior edge of the patch to the margin of the anterior half of the bladder with stay sutures as before (Fig. 9.10).

At the end of the procedure a wound drain is left into the retropubic space and a suprapubic catheter (large enough not to be blocked by the ileal mucus in the urine) is left in the bladder, and this is brought out through the bladder wall and not through the suture line between the bladder and the ileum. Finally, the omentum is brought down to cover the suture lines.

Postoperative management
The wound drain is removed when it stops draining and the suprapubic catheter is clamped on about the eighth postoperative day, by which time the child should be normally active. The parenteral antibiotic regimen is continued for the first 3–5 days and then changed to a low dose prophylactic antibiotic such as trimethoprim, assuming that the urine is sterile at that time.

When the suprapubic catheter is first clamped and the child starts to void spontaneously, a voided volume chart should be kept, noting the time and volume passed and, on two or three occasions, the residual urine volume. Assuming that the child is voiding satisfactorily, the catheter is removed after 24 hours and the patient is discharged home the next day, by which time the suprapubic drain site should have closed. Any excessive urine leakage from this site is dealt with by 24 hours of indwelling urethral catheterization.

Children being managed by intermittent self-catheterization should routinely have an indwelling urethral catheter for a day or two after removal of the suprapubic catheter to allow the suprapubic site to heal before changing to intermittent catheterization.

Three months postoperatively, or thereabouts, the child should be reassessed by VUD to look for any voiding imbalance. If present, it is manifest by a functional obstruction at the level of the distal sphincter mechanism, although the bladder neck may be the site of obstruction (Turner-Warwick 1976) if it has not previously been ablated surgically. The bladder neck is not usually the site of the obstruction because even if it has not been ablated it is usually sufficiently incompetent (particularly in neuropathy) to allow at least partial emptying by straining and because a voiding detrusor contraction of adequate amplitude is commonly retained (Mundy & Stephenson 1985), and this should cause at least 50% emptying. When the

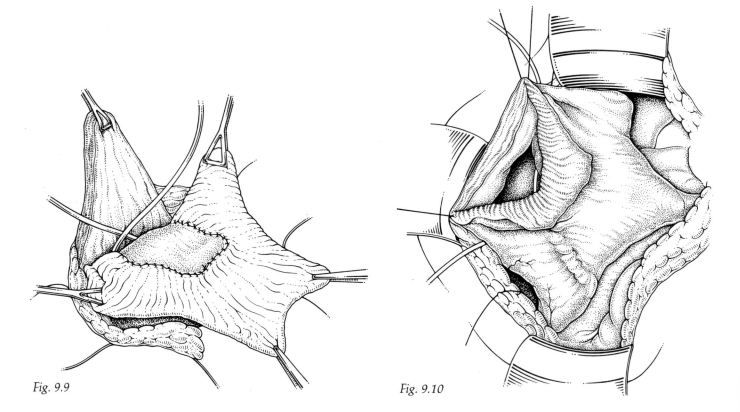

Fig. 9.9

Fig. 9.10

bladder neck is the site of hold-up it is usually because the detrusor contraction is not adequately sustained, giving premature closure of the bladder neck when the bladder is still partly full.

In essence, the difference between those who empty their augmented bladders well and those who do not is the greater ability to empty by straining or expression in the former group and further treatment in the latter group is directed towards improving that means of emptying. This is often achieved simply by letting the child watch his or her own video study to see the residual volume to be eliminated. Otherwise there are two options: either to relax whichever of the two sphincter mechanisms is the objectively demonstrated site of the functional obstruction (usually the distal mechanism) or to use intermittent self-catheterization (Mundy & Stephenson 1985).

The real question, however, is to decide when treatment is necessary at all, and in the asymptomatic child with sterile urine it is probably not necessary. Sphincter rebalancing, either by graded Otis sphincterotomy or by bladder neck incision, whichever is objectively deemed appropriate, or clean intermittent self-catheterization is therefore reserved for the child with persistent postoperative symptoms due to a large residual urine volume or with recurrent urinary tract infections.

The other postoperative complications of augmentation cystoplasty, due to the presence of a gut segment within the urinary tract, are similar to those seen after substitution cystoplasty and are discussed briefly at the end of this chapter.

SUBSTITUTION CYSTOPLASTY

Substitution cystoplasty is used much less commonly and for a wider range of indications than augmentation cystoplasty in children. In some instances the child will have incompetence of the bladder neck and urethral sphincter mechanisms in addition to the bladder problem.

In the absence of such sphincteric incompetence bowel contractility is useful as it facilitates spontaneous voiding. In the presence of sphincteric incompetence, particularly in neuropathy, bowel contractility may be troublesome and cause incontinence, so this must be eliminated by disrupting the bowel musculature by so-called 'detubularization'.

Thus in the absence of sphincteric incompetence an unmodified ('straight' or 'un-detubularized') gut segment is used for bladder substitution. In the presence of sphincteric incompetence, the gut segment is 'detubularized' to form a pouch, recognizing that with a pouch, CISC will be required much more commonly to achieve complete bladder emptying.

The procedure described here for a 'straight' substitution cystoplasty is usually called caecocystoplasty, but in fact the whole of the right colon is used (and some of the transverse colon and the terminal ileum) and so the procedure is more accurately, albeit more clumsily, termed an ileocaeco-colocystoplasty.

A long midline abdominal incision is used. During mobilization of the right side of the colon the middle colic artery will need to be clearly exposed, so the upper end of the incision will need to be high enough to allow this. A point halfway between the umbilicus and the xiphisternum or a little above this is usually sufficient.

The incision is deepened down to the peritoneum, exposing the urachus and the obliterated umbilical ligaments which are ligated together just below the umbilicus where they lie side by side. Above this point the peritoneum is opened in the midline; below this the peritoneum and the underlying fascia are incised just lateral to the obliterated umbilical artery on each side down as far as the point where the artery is crossed by the vas or the round ligament. The peritoneal incision is then extended across from one side to the other along the line of the posterior margin of the bladder. This part of the incision is then deepened to separate the posterior bladder wall, between the two lateral pedicles, from the seminal vesicles in the male and the anterior vaginal wall in the female.

The retropubic space is then widely opened all the way round the front, and including both anterolateral aspects of the bladder, and down to the pelvic floor to expose the anterolateral aspects of the lateral pedicles of the bladder which, having already had their posteromedial aspects exposed by the procedure described in the last paragraph, are thereby clearly defined.

The first stage of the procedure is to perform a subtotal cystectomy, starting with ligation and division of the lateral pedicles. There are four parts of the lateral pedicle which are, from above down, the obliterated umbilical artery, the rest of the superior vesical pedicle, the ureter and the upper part of the inferior vesical pedicle which sweeps up from below the ureter onto the lateral wall of the bladder. These parts should be ligated and divided individually.

The aim of the subtotal cystectomy is to excise all of the bladder except the subureteric part of the trigone. Having ligated the four components of the lateral pedicle, as described above (Fig. 9.11), this is best achieved by first splitting the bladder open in the sagittal plane with diathermy (to reduce bleeding) from the bladder neck anteriorly to the interureteric bar posteriorly. The bladder neck and trigone are then clearly exposed on the inside of the bladder, and each half of the bladder neck and trigone is excised along the margins of the trigone (Fig. 9.12, dotted line), again with diathermy (Figs 9.12, 9.13). There are usually a few bleeding points that need to be secured at the anterior aspect of the bladder neck and at the bases of the lateral pedicles. If the plane between the inter-ureteric region of the bladder base and the seminal vesicles/anterior vaginal wall has not been clearly defined previously, there may be some troublesome bleeding points in this area as well, particularly in girls. These points should be well controlled at this stage as they will be impossible to control with any ease after the cystoplasty segment has been sewn in place.

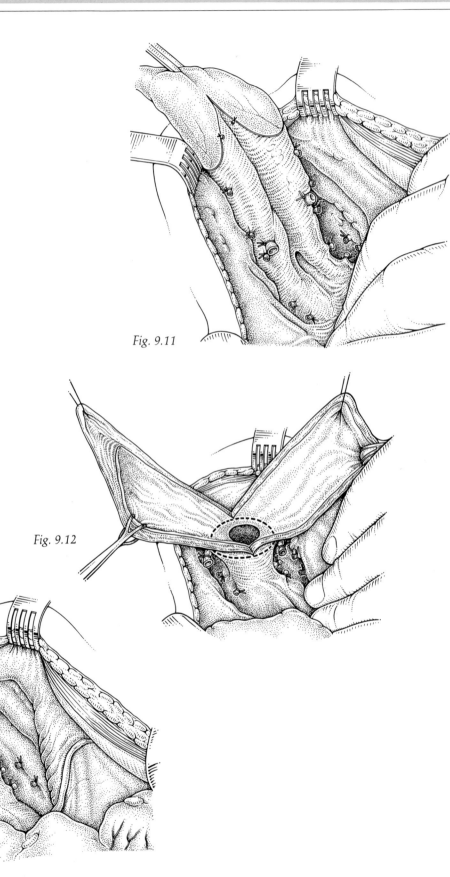

Fig. 9.11

Fig. 9.12

Fig. 9.13

The right side of the colon is then mobilized on its vascular pedicle, starting with an incision in the peritoneum of the right paracolic gutter which is continued around the caecum and terminal ileum below and the hepatic flexure above. This peritoneal incision includes the underlying connective tissue bands that hold the mesocolon onto the posterior abdominal wall, particularly the phrenocolic ligament that runs on the surface of Gerota's fascia to the hepatic flexure. As the mobilization continues, the right colon can be retracted medially, allowing further separation of the right mesocolon and the vessels contained in it from the posterior abdominal wall (Fig. 9.14). As the peritoneal incision is extended around the hepatic flexure, the right lateral limit of the attachment of the omentum to the transverse colon will be encountered. The omentum will need to

be separated from the transverse colon in this area over a length of about 7–10 cm and, assuming that the underlying phrenocolic ligament has been completely divided, this will then allow the right colon and the first part of the transverse colon to be retracted medially to expose the middle colic vessels on their posterior aspect (Fig. 9.15, left). An adequate reflection of the omentum will also expose these vessels on their anterior (peritoneal) aspect, but the vascular anatomy is more easily appreciated from the posterior aspect and a clean exposure of the posterior aspect of the middle colic artery at this stage has the additional advantage of ensuring adequate mobilization of the colonic segment from the underlying duodenum and pancreas, thereby reducing the risk of damage to these structures and to the superior mesenteric vessels.

The key to the vascular supply of the colonic segment is the marginal artery which, at this stage of the operation, can be seen to be supplied by the ileocolic artery below (Fig. 9.15, right), the right branch of the middle colic artery above and the right colic artery between but nearer the ileocolic end (Fig. 9.15, middle). The figure shows the posterior view of these vessels. The sizes of the middle colic, right colic and ileocolic arteries are variable from individual to individual but the marginal artery is constant. It always runs close to the medial aspect of the colon as far as the right branch of the middle colic artery, at which point it runs anatomically up to the bifurcation of the main trunk of the middle colic and down the left branch to continue as the marginal artery again. Hence the importance of an adequate exposure of the middle colic artery.

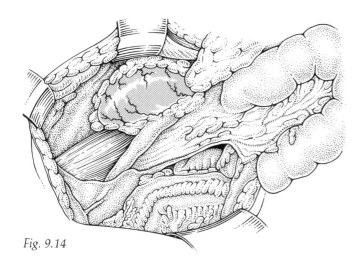

Fig. 9.14

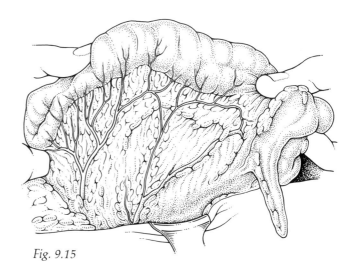

Fig. 9.15

In most cases the best place to divide the colon is between the two branches of the middle colic artery and the best place to divide the blood supply is at the right branch of the middle colic artery, just below the bifurcation.

This will give a colonic segment, supplied by the marginal artery and its arcades and fed by the right colic (if this can be preserved, depending on the anatomy) and ileocolic arteries (Fig. 9.16), of sufficient length to reach down to the bladder remnant with predictable ease (Fig. 9.17) and of sufficient capacity to serve as a substitute bladder (Fig. 9.18). Figure 9.18 shows the cystoplasty segment filled with water to illustrate its capacity.

At the ileocaecal end, the mesenteric vessels are identified, ligated and divided in the usual way to give an ileal tail of about 5–7 cm in length. The isolated ileocaeco-colonic segment is then retracted posteriorly to allow restoration of continuity of the bowel by a two-layer anastomosis of the ileum to the transverse colon in front of the isolated 'cystoplasty' segment.

The cystoplasty segment is then washed out with saline to clear it of any faecal material and to test the competence of the ileocaecal valve.

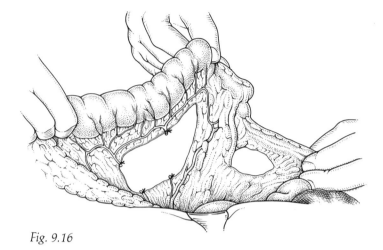

Fig. 9.16

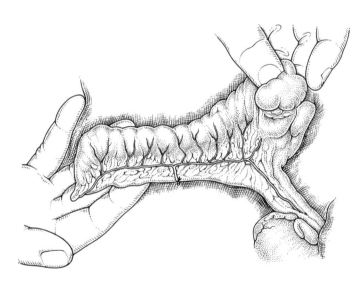

Fig. 9.17

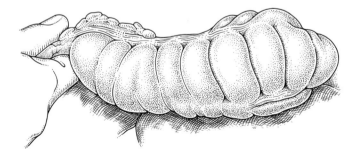

Fig. 9.18

If the ileocaecal valve is sufficiently competent to act as an anti-reflux mechanism, or if an anti-reflux mechanism is thought to be unnecessary or undesirable, the ureters are anastomosed to the ileal tail. First the left ureter is mobilized to above the pelvic brim and then brought across the front of the great vessels, deep to the sigmoid mesocolon, to join to the right ureter side-to-side just above the right common iliac vessels. The cystoplasty segment is then rotated through 180° to put the colonic end into the pelvis and the ileal end in its correct relationship to the common ureteric orifice which is then anastomosed to the ileum with one layer of continuous 3/0 vicryl (Fig. 9.19). The surrounding peritoneum is then tacked to the ileum to retro-peritonealize the uretero-ileal anastomosis.

If the ileocaecal valve is not competent and an anti-refluxing ureteric re-implantation is thought to be necessary, the caecum is opened through an incision into a taenia coli and a tunnel-type of reimplantation is performed of each ureter individually, in the usual way, into the then posterior wall of the caecum, having first rotated the cystoplasty segment into its final position as described above.

This leaves the anastomosis of the colonic end of the cystoplasty segment to the bladder remnant. This is achieved by starting two continuous sutures in the posterior midline and then running one around each side, locking the running stitch at two or three points to prevent a purse-string constriction of the anastomosis (Fig. 9.20). Each bite of the stitch should pick up the full thickness of the colonic wall and both the outer fascial layer of the bladder remnant and the urothelium. In this way the urothelium is splayed out to the outer fascial layer of the bladder remnant, providing a fixed bladder base, and direct mucosal apposition between the two parts of the anastomosis is assured.

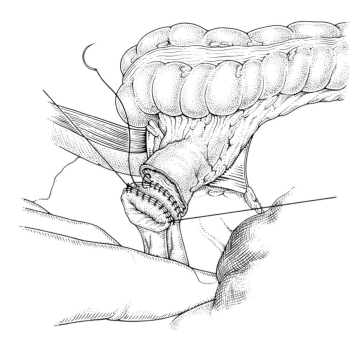

Fig. 9.19

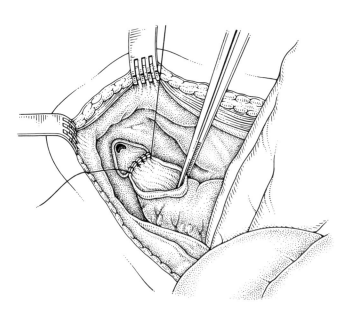

Fig. 9.20

Finally, the defect between the cystoplasty and the right posterolateral wall of the pelvis should be closed to prevent the small bowel prolapsing through it. This is achieved by tacking the peritoneum of the side wall of the pelvis, where it was incised during the course of the subtotal cystectomy, to the colonic segment, taking care not to damage any of the blood vessels in the vascular pedicle.

At the end of the procedure a catheter is left in the cystoplasty bladder through the stump of the appendix (Fig. 9.21). Any large-bore catheter will do, but the author uses a specially designed catheter which has a long section with multiple side holes beyond a 5–10 ml retention balloon (Fig. 9.22). The multiple side holes give a long drainage section to the catheter which makes it less likely to clog up with mucus than an ordinary catheter.

Wound drains are left in the region of the uretero-ileal anastomosis and in the pelvis, the omentum is wrapped around the cystoplasty segment and its upper and lower anastomoses and held in place with a few stitches (Fig. 9.23), and the wound is then closed in the usual way.

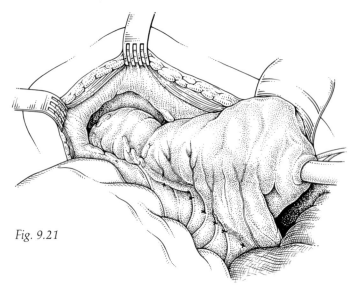

Fig. 9.21

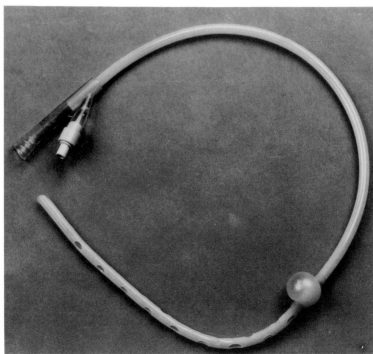

Fig. 9.22

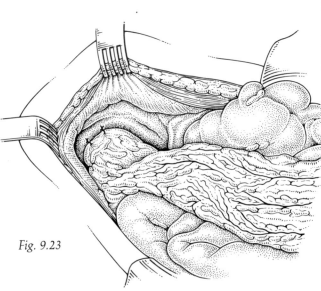

Fig. 9.23

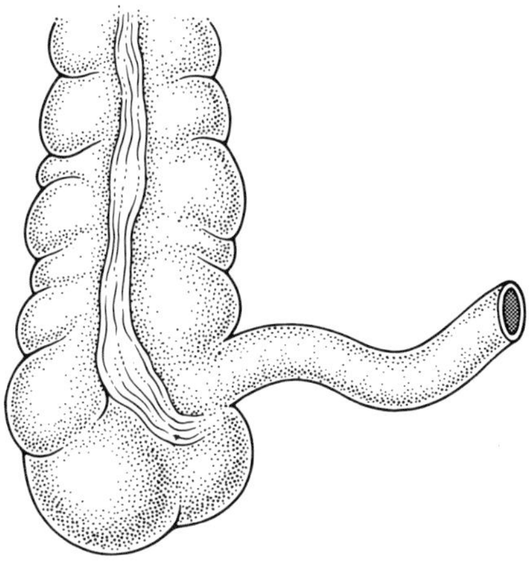

AN ALTERNATIVE SUBSTITUTION CYSTOPLASTY TECHNIQUE—THE ILEOCAECAL POUCH

Troublesome caecocolonic activity is sometimes found after the type of substitution cystoplasty described above, and this may be a cause of incontinence if the child's sphincter mechanisms are unable to contain it. This is particularly so in children with neuropathic sphincter weakness or when a sphincter ablation and implantation of an artificial sphincter have been performed. Colonic activity may in any case be excessive in neuropathy.

For these reasons it is wise to anticipate problems in children with neuropathic hyperreflexia and to modify the cystoplasty technique to ensure a low pressure and acontractile cystoplasty segment. This is achieved by isolating a segment with a longer than usual ileal component that is only 5 cm or so shorter than the caecocolonic part (Fig. 9.24) and then opening up the ileal part and all but the last 5 cm of the colonic part (Fig. 9.25), thereby dividing the circularly orientated smooth muscle in the segment that is presumably responsible for most of the troublesome contractile activity. The ileal segment is then sewn as a patch into the divided colonic segment to produce an ileocaecal pouch (Fig. 9.26). Before closing the pouch, the ureters are reimplanted into the caecum as described above, and after the pouch has been formed, the distal colonic end is sutured to the bladder remnant in the usual way.

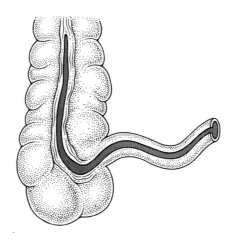

Fig. 9.24

Fig. 9.25

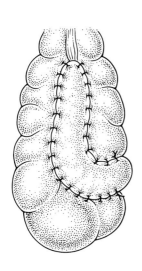

Fig. 9.26a

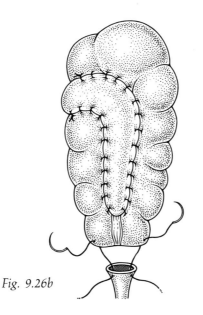

Fig. 9.26b

Postoperative management
This is the same as for augmentation cystoplasty. The only difference is the increased likelihood of voiding difficulties. Although more common with substitution than with augmentation cystoplasty, any voiding difficulty is managed in the same way.

PROBLEMS ASSOCIATED WITH CYSTOPLASTY DUE TO THE PRESENCE OF AN INTESTINAL SEGMENT WITHIN THE URINARY TRACT

Gut continues to function as gut after transposition into the urinary tract, and therefore continues to contract, to secrete mucus and to absorb water and electrolytes.

Gut contractility has already been discussed with reference to 'detubularization'. Problems from mucus secretion are rare in the absence of a voiding imbalance except occasionally in young male children in whom the urethral calibre is small and particularly when CISC is used for emptying. When mucus is a problem, it can be dissolved by instillations of 30 ml of 20% acetyl cysteine.

Fluid absorption by the cystoplasty segment does not usually cause problems, but electrolyte shifts may cause problems of metabolic acidosis and, with colonic segments, hypokalaemia (because of potassium secretion).

All patients with cystoplasties have a metabolic acidosis, usually with respiratory compensation, but this is usually only detectable by arterial blood gas analysis. Only 16% have hyperchloraemia (Nurse & Mundy 1989b). This acidosis may be symptomatic and require oral bicarbonate treatment.

The other major potential problem after cystoplasty is bacterial colonization of the neo-bladder. About 50% of patients with ileocystoplasties and 75% of patients with colocystoplasties develop chronic or recurrent bacteriuria with a mixed growth of organisms. This bacteriuria is associated with a high concentration of urinary nitrosamines which are known carcinogens. The presence of nitrosamines are in turn associated with metaplastic changes in the cystoplasty and the bladder remnant, particularly in colocystoplasties (Nurse & Mundy 1989a). This association is obviously worrying as it suggests that there is a potential for long term malignant change in a cystoplasty similar to that after ureterosigmoidostomy (Leadbetter et al 1979).

Finally, it is important to stress that all of these problems may occur at any stage after operation and lifelong follow-up is therefore important, particularly in view of the possible increased risk of adenocarcinoma developing in the colonic segment after prolonged exposure to urine (Leadbetter et al 1979).

CONCLUSION

Augmentation and substitution cystoplasty are useful and important techniques in the management of a wide range of lower urinary tract problems. To get the best from them requires careful patient selection, appropriate preoperative investigation, attention to detail in the performance of the procedures and careful long-term follow-up.

REFERENCES

Bramble F J 1982 The treatment of adult enuresis and urge incontinence by enterocystoplasty. British Journal of Urology 54: 693–696
Cherney L S 1941 Modified transverse incision for low abdominal operations. Surgery, Gynecology and Obstetrics 72: 92–95
Leadbetter G W, Zickerman P, Pierce E 1979 Ureterosigmoidostomy and carcinoma of the colon. Journal of Urology 121: 732–735
Mundy A R 1985a The neuropathic bladder. In: Postlethwaite R J (ed) Paediatric nephrology. John Wright, Bristol
Mundy A R 1985b The unstable bladder. Urologic Clinics of North America 12: 317–328
Mundy A R 1985c The surgical treatment of refractory detrusor instability. Neurology and Urodynamics 4: 357–365
Mundy A R 1986 Cystoplasty. In: Mundy A R (ed) Current operative surgery — urology. Baillière Tindall, Eastbourne
Mundy A R, Stephenson T P 1984a The urge syndrome. In: Mundy A R, Stephenson T P, Wein A J (eds) Urodynamics: principles, practice and application. Churchill Livingstone, Edinburgh
Mundy A R, Stephenson T P 1984b Selection of patients for implantation of the Brantley Scott artificial urinary sphincter. British Journal of Urology 56: 717–720
Mundy A R, Stephenson T P 1985 'Clam' ileocystoplasty for the treatment of refractory urge incontinence. British Journal of Urology 57: 641–646
Nurse D E, Mundy A R 1989a Assessment of the malignant potential of cystoplasty. British Journal of Urology 64 (in press)
Nurse D E, Mundy A R 1989b Metabolic complications of cystoplasty. British Journal of Urology 63: 165–170
Stephenson T P, Mundy A R 1985 Treatment of the neuropathic bladder by enterocystoplasty and selective sphincterotomy or sphincter ablation and replacement. British Journal of Urology 57: 27–31
Turner-Warwick R T 1976 Cystoplasty. In: Blandy J P (ed) Urology. Blackwell Scientific, Oxford
Turner-Warwick R, Worth P, Milroy E, Duckett J 1974 The suprapubic V incision. British Journal of Urology 46: 39–45

Chapter 10

Ureteric reimplantation for vesico-ureteric reflux

S. Joseph Cohen

Introduction

In the 1950s the problem of vesico-ureteric reflux with urinary infection and resultant pyelonephritis became recognized and many surgical operations to correct reflux were devised. At the time when the efficacy of operative techniques had been proven, physicians showed that similar control of the situation could be obtained by long-term antimicrobial therapy accompanied by the practice of double micturition to reduce residual urine volumes. Extensive controlled double-blind studies are being carried out to compare these two methods, and there are staunch supporters of each.

It is the purpose of this chapter to illustrate the surgical techniques of reimplantation of the ureters and not to be involved in this controversy.

PREOPERATIVE INVESTIGATIONS

Vesico-ureteric reflux was previously only demonstrable by micturating cysto-urethrography (MCU). This procedure is invasive, exposes the child to a fair amount of radiation and is often uncomfortable. Nevertheless, it is still the most effective method of demonstrating the condition. In addition it is the best way to demonstrate the outflow tract, which is essential to differentiate primary reflux from reflux secondary to such outflow obstructions as urethral valves, strictures, duplications, polyps, etc. The newer methods of indirect and direct isotope renography and ultrasonography are being improved and may in the future supercede MCU as the most effective way of making the diagnosis.

Intravenous urography is an essential preoperative investigation for it can statically outline the size, shape, site and number of kidneys and ureters; it also shows the configuration of the pelvis and calyces and the presence or absence of renal scarring. All these factors are of importance in the diagnosis of reflux nephropathy. As with the MCU, the use of radionuclide methods of investigation are now being made more reliable and effective and may in the long term replace the older methods of investigation.

The fact that vesico-ureteric reflux has been demonstrated does not necessarily mean that reimplantation is mandatory; far from it, for the minor degrees of reflux (stages 1 & 2 of Dwoskin & Perlmutter 1973) are best treated by non-surgical means. In grade 5, where there is gross reflux and severe reflux nephropathy, the use of either surgical or medical treatment is unable to reverse the renal pathology and its inevitable consequences.

SURGICAL TECHNIQUES

Since the early 1950s many surgical techniques have been devised for the correction of vesico-ureteric reflux. The earliest was probably that of Hutch (1963) followed by Politano & Leadbetter (1958), Paquin (1959), Glenn & Anderson (1967), Gregoir & Van Regemorter (1964) and Cohen (1975). The techniques are mainly divisible into two groups: first, those where the dissection of the ureter is mainly or entirely intravesical, and second, where the dissection is entirely extravesical, of which Gregoir is the best example.

Recently, the endoscopic injection of Teflon submucosally below and behind the ureteric orifice has been introduced by O'Donnell & Puri (1984), and it appears that the preliminary results are encouraging. Time alone will prove whether this simple procedure is as safe and effective as the more extensive procedures listed above.

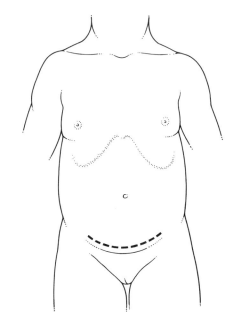

Fig. 10.1

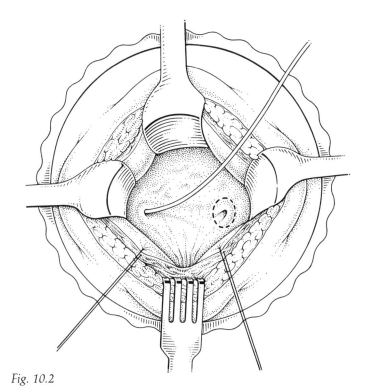

Fig. 10.2

THE OPERATION

Endoscopy should always precede opening of the bladder in order to determine the size, shape and number of the ureteric orifices, to show that there is no outflow obstruction and to confirm that acute cystitis is absent. The latter should persuade the operator to postpone surgery until the inflammation has subsided.

Cohen trans-trigonal technique

A low, transverse, suprapubic incision is made (Fig. 10.1). Its position is such that it is, in later life, hidden in the pubic hair and so will not prevent young girls from wearing bikinis.

After the skin and subcutaneous tissue have been incised, the rectus sheath is exposed. The bladder is approached either by a true Pfannenstiel incision, i.e. transverse division of the rectus sheath with separation of the rectus muscles, or by dividing the sheath vertically between the recti and then separating them. When this has been done, vesical stay sutures are inserted and between them the bladder is opened vertically or by a T incision. A Denis Browne ring retractor is inserted as illustrated in Figure 10.2. A swab inserted under the apical retractor blade facilitates the exposure. The ureteric orifices are carefully examined as regards site, size, number, shape and the length of tunnels. A fine infant feeding tube is inserted up the ureter and fixed by a fine Dexon or catgut suture, as shown on the patient's right side in the figure. A circumferential incision is then made around the orifice, as shown on the patient's left side.

Dissection of the ureter is now carried out. The incision is deepened, carefully dividing the muscle fibres that fix the ureter to the bladder trigone (Fig. 10.3). It is wise to commence just below the orifice and, once the plane is found between the ureter and bladder musculature, this is progressively developed around the ureter until the latter is completely freed. Great care must be taken not to dissect too close to the ureter for fear of damaging its blood supply or its musculature. The peritoneum, which almost surrounds the ureter, must be carefully teased away using a small pledget. In male patients the vas deferens may lie close to this point and accidental damage must be carefully avoided.

The ureter is now free and ready for reimplantation. In the majority of cases the opposite ureter is freed in the same way and reimplantation may commence. The dissection of the ureter may have enlarged its vesical hiatus to such an extent that it should be narrowed with one, two or three 3/0 or 4/0 Dexon sutures in order to prevent the subsequent formation of a bladder diverticulum. The submucosal tunnel is then constructed; a point is selected above and perhaps a little lateral to the opposite ureteric orifice. An incision in the mucosa is made and, after inserting its closed blades, a pair of scissors is advanced under the mucosa by an opening and closing movement (Fig.

10.4). This is continued until the ureter is reached. The tunnel should be a gentle curve, a prolongation of the entrance of the ureter into the bladder. Care must be taken as one approaches the midline for it is here that the mucosa is easily buttonholed. This can be best avoided by placing a pair of Allis forceps just lateral to the commencement of the tunnel and, by gently retracting these laterally, the posterior bladder wall can be straightened and the problem averted. The new tunnel must be wide enough to comfortably hold the ureter, and long enough to prevent reflux. The minimal length is two to three times the ureteric diameter.

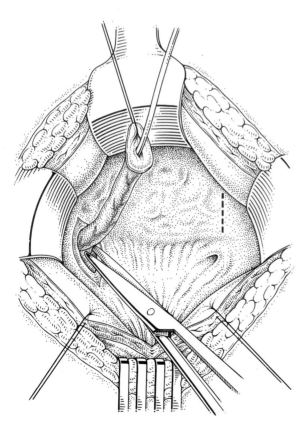

Fig. 10.3

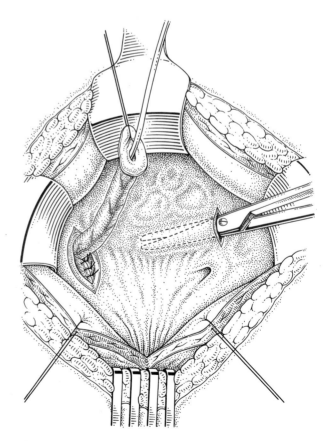

Fig. 10.4

The ureter is now gently threaded through its new tunnel (Fig. 10.5). This is best accomplished by passing a pair of forceps into the tunnel, grasping the stay suture and drawing the ureter into place, taking care not to twist or kink it in the process.

The cuff of the ureter is then sutured into position (Fig. 10.6). Firstly a 3/0 Dexon suture is inserted through the full thickness of the cuff and also through a full thickness of bladder muscle. This prevents the ureter from retracting. Next, three or four 5/0 Dexon sutures are inserted, joining the bladder and ureteric mucosae. The incision in the mucosa of the original orifice is closed with fine Dexon sutures. Many surgeons do not believe in retaining this cuff of ureteric mucosa, but if it has not been devascularized, traumatized or the site of stenosis, this author believes that it is worth preserving. If any doubt exists, then the terminal part of the ureter should be excised.

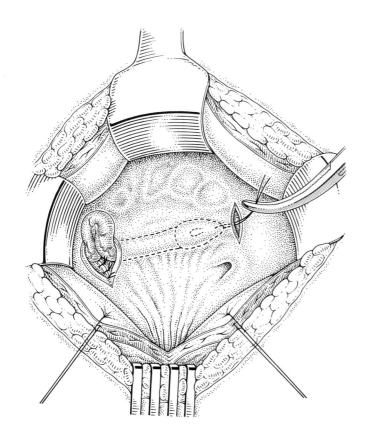

Fig. 10.5

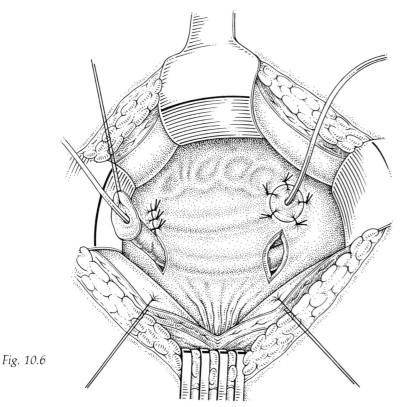

Fig. 10.6

Bilateral reimplantation

The dissection of both ureters having been carried out as mentioned above, the two ureters are held and assessed as to which would sit most comfortably in the upper tunnel. If both seem equally well suited, then this author tends to use the upper tunnel for the ureter that has the more severe degree of reflux. The second tunnel is then constructed by the same technique as above. Its position is below the tunnel already made, and goes from the ureteric entrance to the orifice of the opposite side. The ureter is threaded through in the same manner and similarly fixed in its new position. In the very young, where the intertrigonal distance is short, the tunnel may be extended through this orifice to a point farther lateral and fixed there. Some surgeons have used a single tunnel for both ureters and have had no trouble from this, but on theoretical grounds the two ureters may adhere to one another and this author still prefers to use separate tunnels.

Bladder closure

Having made sure that the ureters are lying comfortably in their new tunnels and are well vascularized to their tips, the swab is removed from the bladder; fine infant feeding tubes are inserted up the reimplanted ureters, and bladder closure is carried out. The mucosa should be closed with a continuous fine Dexon or catgut suture (4/0 or 5/0). The bladder muscle is closed with interrupted 2/0 or 3/0 Dexon or catgut sutures, with a Malecot catheter left in situ for bladder drainage. In girls, one may use a Foley transurethral catheter. A drain is inserted retropubically and the muscles and fasciae closed with 2/0 or 3/0 Dexon or catgut. The skin is closed with a continuous subcuticular 4/0 Dexon suture.

Reimplantation in duplex systems

Ureteric duplication may be complete or incomplete. Where it is complete, the lower moiety ureter is the one that is laterally placed and often incompetent. The two ureters are often very closely adherent and may even share a common musculature and blood supply. This necessitates dissection of the two ureters as a single unit, without attempting to separate one from the other. The technique would therefore be exactly the same as that illustrated in Figures 10.4 and 10.5.

CONCLUSIONS

Reimplantation of the ureters is recognized as a reliable method of correcting vesico-ureteric reflux. Its efficacy has been proven over the last three decades and one should expect to achieve success in virtually all cases. The complication rate is also continuously being reduced, and one should expect this in only 1–4% of cases. Obstructive complications are more common in those cases where there was originally gross dilatation of the ureters or where the bladder was thickened and trabeculated due to a neurogenic abnormality or previous outflow obstruction.

REFERENCES

Cohen S J 1975 Ureterozystoneostomie: ein neue antireflux technik. Aktuelle Urologie 6: 1–6
Dwoskin J Y, Perlmutter A D 1973 Vesico-ureteric reflux in children: a computerised review. Journal of Urology 109: 888–890
Glenn J F, Anderson E E 1967 Distal tunnel ureteral reimplantation. Journal of Urology 97: 623–626
Gregoir W, Van Regemorter G 1964 Le reflux vesico-ureteral congenital. Urologia Internationalis 18: 12
Hutch J A 1963 Ureteric advancement operation: anatomy, technique and early results. Journal of Urology 89: 180–184
O'Donnell B, Puri P 1984 Treatment of vesico-ureteric reflux by endoscopic injection of Teflon. British Medical Journal 289: 7–9
Paquin A J Jr 1959 Uretero-vesical anastomosis: the description and evaluation of a technique. Journal of Urology 82: 573–583
Politano V A, Leadbetter W F 1958 An operative technique for the correction of vesico-ureteral reflux. Journal of Urology 79: 932–941

Chapter 11

Standard orchidopexy techniques for undescended testes

J. H. Johnston

Introduction

It is accepted that an undescended testis should be placed in the scrotum during childhood in order to promote its spermatogenic potential and also, but with much less confidence, to lessen the likelihood of the later development of a neoplasm.

There have been differing opinions as to the preferred method of obtaining testicular descent. Hormone treatment was introduced in the 1930s and, at first, excellent results were recorded. Later, it became clear that the successes were mainly in normal boys with retractile testes. More recent series in which retractile testes were excluded have reported a failure rate of 81% in boys under 3 years of age and of 55% in boys aged 3–5 years with the use of gonadotrophic hormone (Garagoni et al 1982). Illig et al (1977), employing luteinizing hormone-releasing hormone, stated that therapy led to complete descent in 38% of testes, to an improved position in 28% and to no change in 19%. Hormone therapy during childhood induces a degree of precocious puberty with the possibility of premature epiphyseal· fusion, and there have been reports of degenerative changes in the retained testis following its use (Charny & Wolgin 1957). The method is clearly indicated in the patient with hypogonadotrophic hypo-gonadism, and some surgeons have employed it preoperatively hopefully to facilitate an anticipated difficult orchidopexy. However, as a definitive form of treatment in the common situation of a cryptochid boy without endocrinopathy, hormones are effective in only a minority of cases, they carry the possibility of causing undesirable side-effects, and they have no advantages over orchidopexy in competent hands.

The optimal timing of orchidopexy has been disputed. Electron micro-scopy studies have indicated that degenerative changes begin in the undescended testis within the first 2 years of life (Mininberg et al 1982), and modern opinion has favoured orchidopexy at 2 years of age or even earlier. However, there is no doubt that the operation is much easier, and therefore safer, for the testis, in the somewhat older boy. Thorup et al (1984) recorded that their clinical results were significantly better when orchidopexy was deferred until later childhood. The surgeon must make his own judgement concerning timing according to his own experience. The decision is commonly made for him when, as is often the case, the patient presents only after his first school examination aged 5–6 years.

In bilateral cases both testes may be dealt with at the same operative session, but if there is any doubt about the outcome of the first orchidopexy, as will almost invariably be the case with intra-abdominal testes (see below), an interval of some months is advisable since the result achieved on the first side may influence the management of the opposite testis.

The operative technique depends on the position of the testis.

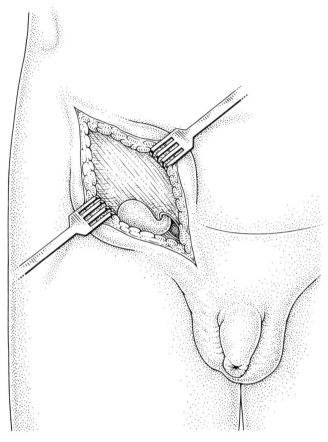

Fig. 11.1

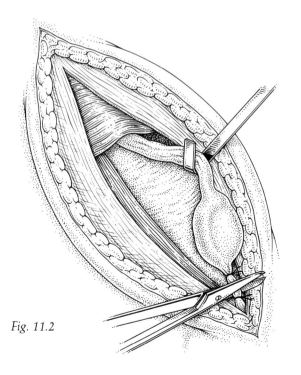

Fig. 11.2

INGUINAL APPROACH

This method is applicable to the majority of cases of testicular undescent where the testis lies in the inguinal canal or is palpable outside the superficial inguinal ring.

An oblique incision is made over the inguinal canal and deepened to expose the external oblique aponeurosis, the superficial ring and, often, the emerging testis within its fascial coverings (Fig. 11.1). As shown, the testis commonly lies ectopically lateral to the ring in the superficial inguinal pouch.

The external oblique aponeurosis is divided upwards and laterally from the ring. The cremaster muscle is incised longitudinally and the spermatic cord and the testis are delivered into the wound (Fig. 11.2). The gubernacular remains below the testis are divided between ligatures; during this procedure care must be taken to avoid injury to the globus minor of the epididymis or to the vas deferens since these structures commonly lie lower than the body of the testis.

The tunica vaginalis is opened and probed proximally to determine whether or not there is a patent processus vaginalis. If there is, the sac is divided just above the testis and dissected from the cord to the level of the deep inguinal ring where it is ligated and excised (Fig. 11.3). An incomplete hernial sac is rare with testicular undescent but a pseudo-sac can be produced by traction on the spermatic cord during mobilization; it is readily freed from the cord and does not need to be excised.

Further descension of the cord reveals the suspensory spermatic fascial ligament of Denis Browne (1949), which extends upwards and laterally through the deep inguinal ring. Division of this band (Fig. 11.4) is the procedure which achieves the most significant cord lengthening; often, as the cord descends it can be incised at more than one level.

The above measures often suffice to let the testis come to the scrotum. If not, the fascia transversalis forming the posterior wall of the inguinal canal can be incised from the inner edge of the deep ring (Fig. 11.5). The cord can then move medially, eliminating its slight angulation at the ring. It is not necessary to divide the inferior epigastric vessels, which are readily displaced.

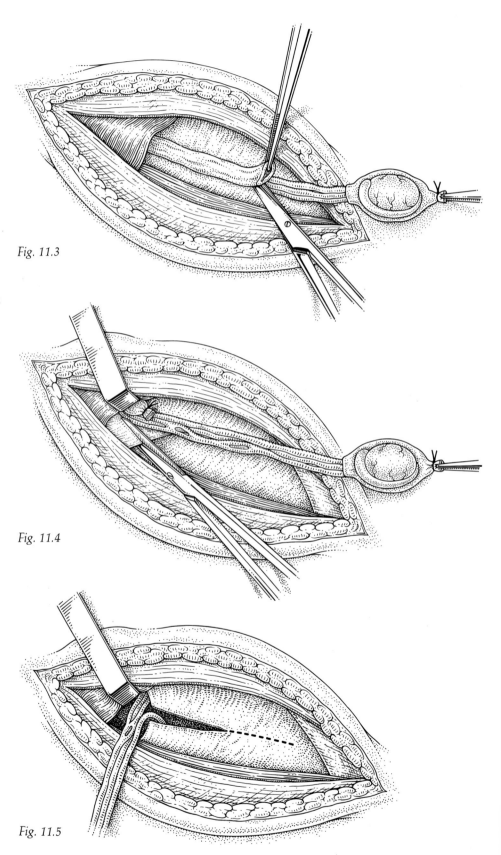

Fig. 11.3

Fig. 11.4

Fig. 11.5

If sufficient cord lengthening is not obtained by these manoeuvres, the abdominal incision can be extended upwards and laterally and, with suitable retraction, the spermatic vessels and the vas can be further freed from their surroundings. Often, however, this intra-abdominal dissection achieves very little extra length. A testis that will still not reach the scrotum can be fixed by suture at its lowest position and then explored some 6 months later when re-mobilization is often successful in obtaining enough cord length. The second stage of the operation is facilitated if the testis and cord are wrapped in a thin Silastic sheet at the end of the first stage in order to prevent them adhering to the surrounding scar tissue.

Fixation of the testis in the scrotum
A variety of techniques have been described for this purpose. If the testis can be brought easily to the scrotal fundus, virtually any method will suffice, but none can compensate for insufficient cord length. The following method is generally applicable:

A finger is passed down from the inguinal incision to stretch the hemi-scrotum (Fig. 11.6). A small skin incision is made over the finger tip.

A subcutaneous pouch is formed by scissors dissection (Fig. 11.7).

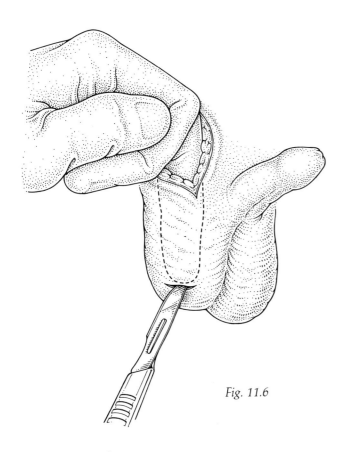

Fig. 11.6

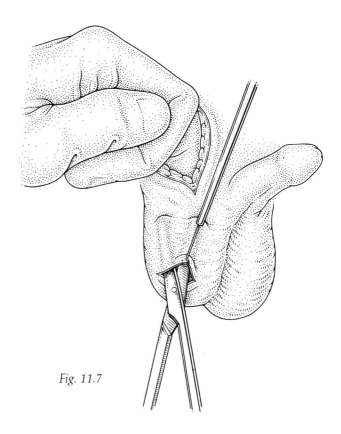

Fig. 11.7

A small incision is made in the scrotal fascia through which an artery forceps is passed to grasp the stump of the gubernaculum (Fig. 11.8).

The testis is drawn into the subcutaneous pouch. The incision in the fascia is narrowed around the emerging spermatic cord to prevent the testis retracting upwards. The groin and scrotal incisions are closed (Fig. 11.9).

Fowler–Stephens technique
Fowler & Stephens (1959) confirmed that the vasal vessels alone can often adequately vascularize the testis so that division of the spermatic vessels may be safely carried out when they are too short to let the testis come to the scrotum.

Fowler & Stephens described their technique as being especially applicable to the case in which the vas deferens, with its accompanying vessels, forms a loop below the testis. A vascular clamp is placed on the spermatic vessels above the communications between them (Fig. 11.10) and the vasal vessels and the effect on the testis observed. If uncertainty exists concerning the adequacy of the testicular blood supply, one of the subtunical vessels on the testis can be divided to allow the quality of the bleeding to be seen. When the vascularity of the testis is assured, the spermatic vessels are divided between ligatures. Division of one or two of the vascular arcades crossing the loop then allows the vas to be straightened sufficiently to allow the testis to reach the scrotum. Great care is needed to prevent injury to the vasal vessels, particularly during the freeing of a hernial sac.

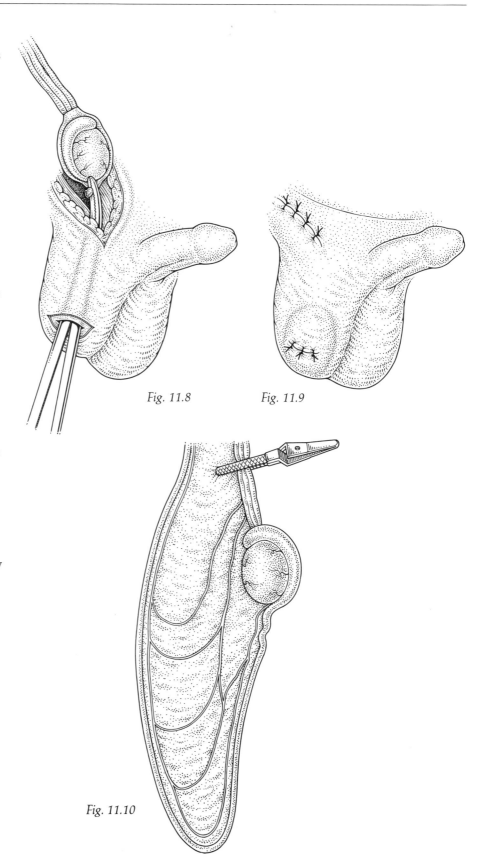

Fig. 11.8   Fig. 11.9

Fig. 11.10

THE HIGH INTRA-ABDOMINAL TESTIS

The classic example of this form of cryptorchidism is encountered bilaterally in boys with the prune belly syndrome. Each testis is suspended within the peritoneal cavity in a mesentery at the postero-lateral aspect of the pelvic brim. The spermatic vessels are very short but the vas and its accompanying vessels are correspondingly long. For reasons already discussed, orchidopexy should be performed one side at a time.

The peritoneal cavity is opened through an oblique, muscle-cutting incision in the iliac fossa (right in the drawing) and the testis in its mesentery is delivered into the wound (Fig. 11.11). The spermatic vessels superiorly, the gubernaculum inferiorly and the vas with its accompanying vessels centrally are recognized. Vascular clamps are applied to the spermatic vessels above the communications with the vasal vessels and to the gubernaculum, and the effect on the testis is observed. As already described, doubt concerning testicular vascularity can be resolved by division of one of the subtunical vessels.

If the testis remains well vascularized, the spermatic vessels and the gubernaculum are divided between ligatures at the levels of clamping (Fig. 11.12). A strip of peritoneum is left attached to the vas in order to avoid damaging the vasal vessels; the vas may need to be gently freed from the bladder wall in order to obtain sufficient extra length. The inguinal canal in such cases is non-existent. To bring the testis to the scrotum an artery forceps is passed through a scrotal incision, as shown in Figure 11.8, and guided obliquely through the abdominal parietes in the inguinal region. The testis is drawn down, care being taken to avoid torsion of the vasal pedicle, and fixed in a subcutaneous pouch, as in Figure 11.9. Closure of the peritoneum around the emerging vas at the groin is performed *secundum artem* and the abdominal and scrotal incisions are sutured.

Ransley (1984) has described a two-staged modification of the above technique which is safer for the testis. At the first stage, ligation of the spermatic vessels is performed. Some months later, following the establishment of an assured collateral testicular circulation through the vasal vessels, the second stage is carried out as described.

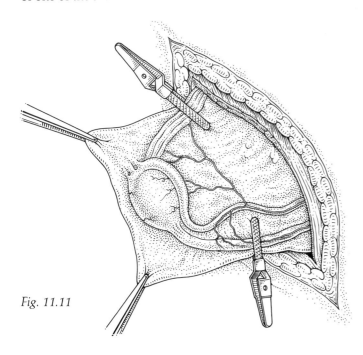

Fig. 11.11

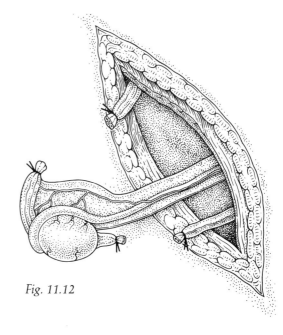

Fig. 11.12

THE IMPOSSIBLE ORCHIDOPEXY

There has been no uniformity of opinion concerning the management of the boy with bilateral cryptorchidism in whom neither testis can be made to reach the scrotum with an assured blood supply. Concern about the increased risk of neoplasia in the retained testis in adult life may persuade the surgeon to advocate bilateral orchidectomy during childhood to be followed by hormone replacement at the age of puberty. However, in the male who is congenitally anorchic or rendered so at an early age, exogenous testosterone therapy fails to produce normal virilization as regards growth of hair on the face, axillae and pubis and it cannot be relied upon to induce long-term sexual potency, although early effects are often very encouraging. The present author's preference is to preserve at least one testis so that its hormonal function will be retained and, if possible, to place it in a subcutaneous position in the groin where it is easily palpable so that possible malignant change can be detected early. It must be remembered that cancer in an undescended testis, although reportedly some 30 times greater than average, is still an uncommon lesion as compared with tumours in other organs. In the Merseyside region of England during 1973, the incidence of testicular tumour per 100 000 males was 1.7 whereas the corresponding figures for cancer of the rectum, bladder, prostate, colon, stomach and bronchus were 18.3, 22.5, 23.4, 25.3, 35.0 and 123.0 respectively. Tibbs (1961) estimated that a male with an undescended testis carries a risk of only one chance in 66 of developing a testicular neoplasm during an adult life span of 50 years.

REFERENCES

Browne D 1949 Treatment of undescended testicle. Proceedings of the Royal Society of Medicine 42: 643

Charny C W, Wolgin, W A 1957 Cryptorchism. Cassell, London

Fowler R, Stephens F D 1959 The role of testicular vascular anatomy in the salvage of high undescended testes. Australian and New Zealand Journal of Surgery 29: 92

Garagoni J M, Job J C, Canlrobe P, Chaussain J L 1982 Results of early treatment of cryptorchism with human chorionic gonadotrophin. Journal of Pediatrics 101: 923

Illig R, Kollman F, Barkenstein M et al 1977 Treatment of cryptorchidism by intranasal synthetic luteinising hormone releasing hormone. Lancet ii: 518

Mininberg D T, Rodger J C, Bedford J M 1982 Ultrastructural evidence of onset of testicular pathological conditions in cryptorchid human testes within first year of life. Journal of Urology 128: 782

Ransley P G 1984 Preliminary ligation of the gonadal vessels prior to orchidopexy for the intra-abdominal testicle. A staged Fowler–Stephens procedure. World Journal of Urology 2: 266

Thorup J, Kvist N, Lasen P et al 1984 Clinical results of early and late operative correction of undescended testes. British Journal of Urology 56: 322

Tibbs D J 1961 Unilateral absence of the testes—eight cases of true monorchism. British Journal of Surgery 48: 601

Chapter 12

Microvascular orchidopexy for high undescended testes

A. Bianchi

Introduction

It is well accepted that normal spermatogenesis will only occur if the testis lies in a scrotal environment. Mengel et al (1981), Hadziselimovic (1977) and others have shown that those testes which remain undescended undergo a progressive loss of spermatogonia and marked alteration in tubular structure commencing after the second year of life. Indeed, testes that have not reached the scrotum by the fourth year of life will not achieve normal spermatogenesis after puberty. The higher the testis is retained, the more dysgenetic are its morphological characteristics. Furthermore, the incidence of malignancy is maximal for these organs and appears to be related to their dysgenetic content and also their position (Hausfeld & Schrandt 1965).

Controversy still exists regarding the normality of the high inguinal and intra-abdominal testis at birth, and hence its potential for spermatogenesis. Although a greater proportion of organs retained in such high positions are intrinsically abnormal, most demonstrate varying numbers of spermatogonia. Leydig cell function is not similarly affected and is usually retained, so the majority of high testes will produce sufficient testosterone to induce virilization.

Orchidopexy has been shown to be associated with improved testicular growth and spermatogenesis, and hence a higher fertility rate (Ludwig & Potempa 1975). However, the effect of early orchidopexy with retention of a full blood supply on the subsequent development of the intra-abdominal and high inguinal testis remains unclear. Present-day microvascular techniques have made full revascularization a reliable immediate possibility; however, until further information becomes available, the management of high inguinal and intra-abdominal testes should not be different from those in lower positions.

INDICATIONS FOR ORCHIDOPEXY

The indications for orchidopexy for high inguinal and intra-abdominal testes differ only in emphasis from those in lower positions. Orchidopexy aims to:

a.   Afford the testis the best possible chance for maximal spermatogenesis and hence improved fertility;
b.   Preserve endogenous hormone production;
c.   Reduce the incidence of complications such as torsion, inguinal hernia and psychological disturbance;
d.   Reduce the risk of malignancy and allow early detection of neoplastic change by easy self-examination.

TIMING OF ORCHIDOPEXY

The incidence of testicular undescent in the mature newborn infant is between 1.8 and 4%, but falls to 0.7% by the end of the first year of life (Scorer 1964). More recently, Jackson et al (1986) have reported an incidence of 1.58% at 3 months which, when compared with 0.96% in 1960, indicates a 65% increase in the cryptorchidism rate over two decades. True undescent after one year is always pathological. Mengel et al (1981), Hedinger (1979), Hadziselimovic (1977) and others have demonstrated marked structural alterations and a progressive and rapid loss of spermatogonia in the undescended testis after the second year of life.

Ludwig & Potempa (1975) noted maximal fertility rates when orchidopexy was performed before the end of the second year of life. Furthermore, Martin & Menck (1975) have indicated that testes which have been brought into the scrotum early show less likelihood of late malignancy.

There would seem to be no justification therefore for delaying orchidopexy beyond the end of the second year of life, particularly since the child's age and testicular vessel size are no barrier to microvascular anastomosis.

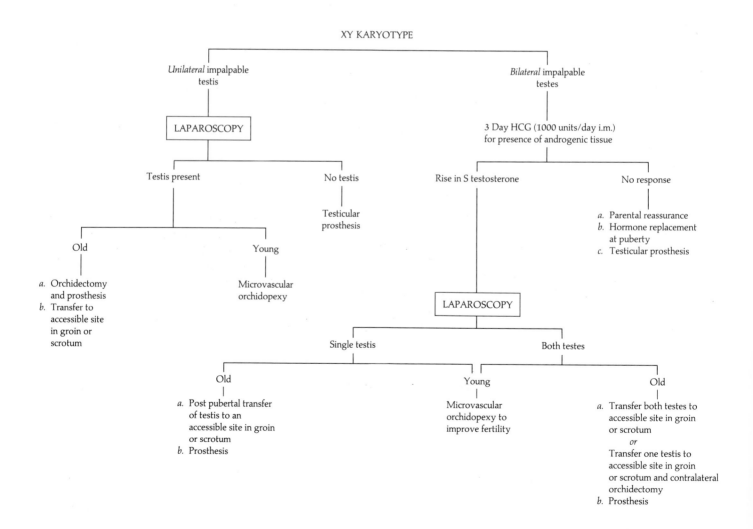

OPERATIVE OPTIONS FOR INTRA-ABDOMINAL TESTES

The short vascular pedicle of the high inguinal and intra-abdominal testis does not lengthen sufficiently even after maximal retroperitoneal mobilization to allow the testis to reach the scrotum.

Multistage orchidopexy (Corkery 1975, Levitt et al 1978) or reliance on the vessels of the vas (Fowler & Stephens 1959) or the surrounding tissues for testicular revascularization have been proposed but have not given consistently satisfactory results. The reliability of microvascular techniques in ensuring anastomotic patency in vessels under 1 mm diameter has made possible scrotal placement of the high inguinal and intra-abdominal testis with an immediate and full blood supply. Microvascular anastomosis of the testicular to the inferior epigastric vessels thus forms an integral part of orchidopexy for such high organs and is the preferred form of management.

MANAGEMENT OF THE IMPALPABLE TESTIS

The factors influencing the management of high undescended and impalpable testes are similar both for unilateral and bilateral cryptorchids. The location and quality of each testis, vascular pedicle and vas, and the age of the child in relation to spermatogenesis and testicular malignancy, form the basis of management and are outlined in the flow diagram (opposite).

It is noteworthy that the incidence of unilateral monorchia is 3%, and of bilateral anorchia is 0.6%. It follows therefore that it is always important to locate an impalpable testis. Of the several investigations proposed, laparoscopy provides maximal definite information regarding testes, vascular pedicles and vasa, with minimal morbidity. All other procedures are less informative and, such as angiography, may well be hazardous. Surgical exploration of the groin should be avoided since it disrupts tissue planes and may damage the inferior epigastric vessels.

LONG-TERM FOLLOW-UP

The increased incidence of malignancy in high undescended and intra-abdominal testes makes long-term follow-up into adulthood essential. Once the testis has been placed in a palpable position, the patient should be taught the art of self-examination. Late orchidectomy, at around 30 years of age, should be given serious consideration.

EQUIPMENT AND REQUIREMENTS

The operating microscope
Magnification is essential for anastomosis of vessels under 1 mm in diameter. Foot pedal control for focus and zoom and an XY coupling are important features and are incorporated in the Zeiss OPMI 6SDFC XY operating microscope. Optical loupe magnification ($\times 3 - \times 4$) is helpful in large vessel dissection but is inadequate for microanastomosis.

Microsurgical instruments
Instruments suitable for microvascular procedures include:

a. Microvascular scissors
b. Jewellers forceps no. 5 or 3
c. Vessel dilator
d. Microneedle holder
e. Graded microvascular clamps and applicator suitable for arteries and veins from 0.3 mm to 1.5 mm in diameter
f. Bipolar diathermy with fine microforceps
g. Sutures: 10/0 or 11/0 non-reactive monofilament suture on the smallest atraumatic needle (3.75 mm, 75 µm), e.g. Ethicon W2870

Anticoagulants
Local washing of vessel ends with a heparin solution, 10 units/ml, is all that is required. Systemic anticoagulants or drugs affecting platelet function such as aspirin or dipyridamole are unnecessary.

Anaesthesia
General anaesthesia with muscle relaxation is needed. Otherwise, routine supportive and monitoring procedures are as for any 4-hour procedure.

SURGICAL TECHNIQUE

Reliable anastomotic patency in vessels under 1 mm in diameter is largely dependent on a high degree of technical skill achieved and maintained in the laboratory by the microvascular surgeon. Only one testis should be transferred at each operation.

THE OPERATION

The child is positioned supine on a heating blanket on the operating table to allow access for the operating microscope and a comfortable position for the surgeon and assistant. A urethral catheter may be passed for the duration of the operation and removed subsequently. Drapes are applied, providing access to the loin, groin and scrotum.

The incision (Fig. 12.1)
A groin incision is made in a skin crease above the inguinal ligament, extending upwards and laterally towards the loin.

Opening the inguinal canal (Fig. 12.2)
The external oblique aponeurosis is incised in the line of its fibres and the inguinal canal opened. The gubernacular structures and processus vaginalis may be identifiable in this plane and are a guide to the internal inguinal ring.

The inferior epigastric vessels (Fig. 12.3)
The dissection is carried through the internal oblique and transversus abdominis to identify the inferior epigastric vessels as they pass beneath the internal inguinal ring. The vessels are carefully dissected free, extending upwards beneath the lateral edge of the rectus abdominis; vessel length and a better lumenal diameter matching that of the testicular vessels are thus achieved. Several muscular branches require ligation or coagulation with bipolar diathermy. Optical loupe magnification is helpful during this procedure.

The vessels are clamped with graded microvascular clamps and divided. The vessel ends are washed with heparin solution (10 units/ml).

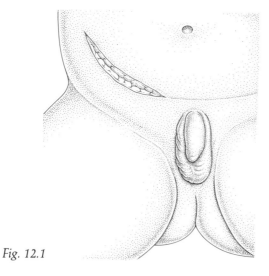

Fig. 12.1

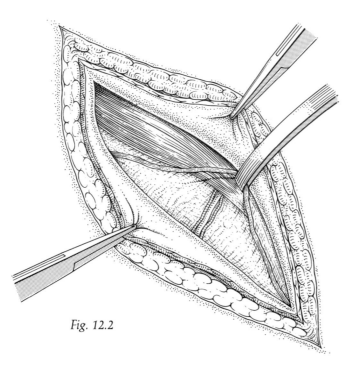

Fig. 12.2

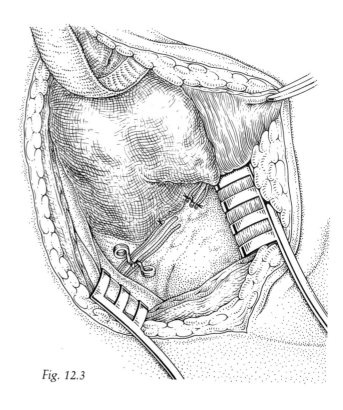

Fig. 12.3

The testis, testicular vessels and vas
(Fig. 12.4)

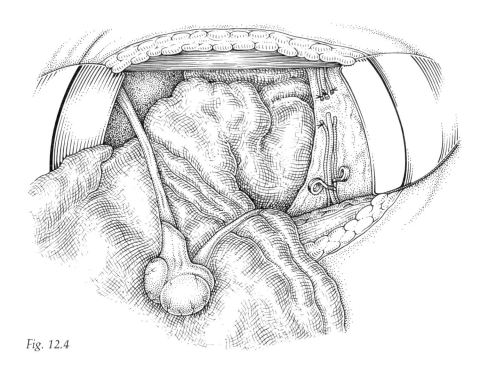

Fig. 12.4

The testis. The peritoneal cavity is opened at the internal inguinal ring and the testis delivered out of the abdomen by severing all its peritoneal attachments. The peritoneum is closed, obliterating the processus vaginalis, and all further dissection is undertaken retroperitoneally.

The testicular vessels. The testicular vessels are carefully mobilized by blunt retroperitoneal dissection towards their origin and beyond the confluence of the venous plexus to form one or two veins. Communicating veins between the testicular venous plexus and the perinephric fat require ligation or coagulation with bipolar diathermy.

A second higher incision is not required, since access to the testicular pedicle is adequate.

The vas. Finger dissection along the vas deep into the pelvis is usually sufficient. It may occasionally be necessary to pass the testis beneath the lateral umbilical ligament to allow sufficient tension-free length on the vas for the testis to reach the scrotum.

Formation of an extradartos pouch
(Fig. 12.5)
A path is opened with a finger between the groin incision and the ipsilateral scrotal compartment. A skin crease incision is made in the scrotal skin and a pocket is formed by blunt dissection between the skin and the dartos muscle. A communicating buttonhole incision is made through the dartos muscle.

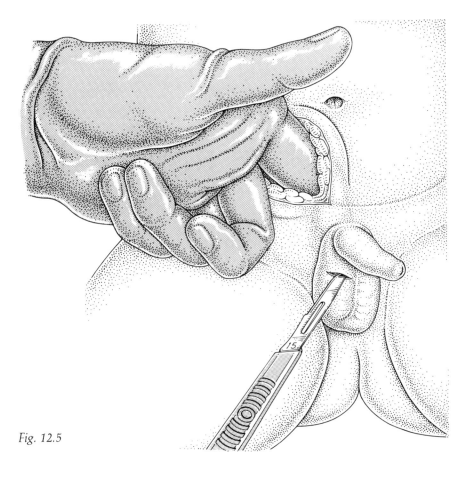

Fig. 12.5

Testicular transfer to the scrotum
(Fig. 12.6)
The testicular vessels are divided close to their origin and the ends washed with heparin solution. Back bleeding, if any, from the testicular vessels is controlled with graded microvascular clamps. The testis is passed into the extradartos pouch, and may be kept cool with a cold saline swab.

Preparation of vessel ends and vascular anastomosis (Fig. 12.7)
Under magnification with the operating microscope, the cut ends of the testicular and inferior epigastric vessels are trimmed back, removing any traumatized areas, and the adventitia dissected away. On no account should the intima be damaged by handling or inserting instruments or cannulae. Testicular perfusion is unnecessary and may be hazardous.

End-to-end anastomoses are performed between the testicular artery (approximately 0.5 mm diameter) and the inferior epigastric artery (approximately 1 mm diameter), and the testicular vein (approximately 1.2 mm diameter) and an inferior epigastric vein (0.8–1 mm diameter). Interrupted sutures of 10/0 nylon on a 3.75 mm, 75 µm, needle accurately appose undamaged intimal surfaces and allow for eventual growth at the anastomosis. Sufficient sutures are inserted to achieve a leak-proof anastomosis.

Overcoming vessel diameter discrepancy (Fig. 12.8)
During end-to-end anastomosis, a spatulate incision on the testicular artery overcomes the discrepancy in lumenal diameter. Alternatively, an end-to-side anastomosis to the inferior epigastric artery achieves the same goal.

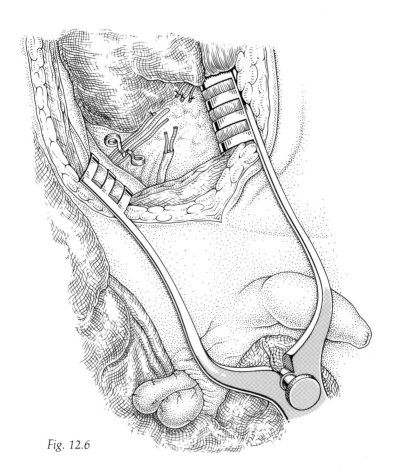

Fig. 12.6

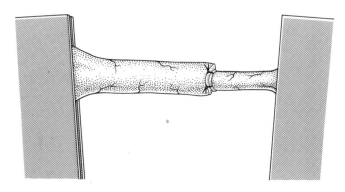

Fig. 12.7

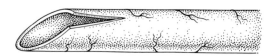

Fig. 12.8

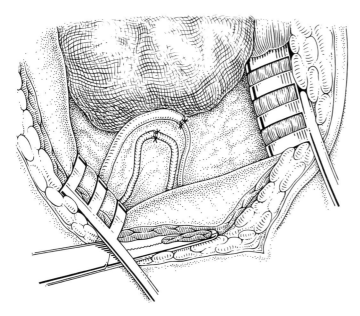

Fig. 12.9

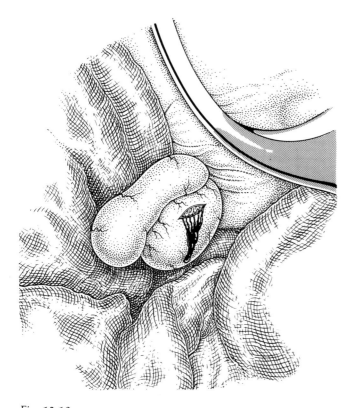

Fig. 12.10

Testicular revascularization (Fig. 12.9)
On completion of both anastomoses all microvascular clamps are removed, ending with that on the inferior epigastric artery. The anastomoses should be carefully observed but left undisturbed for at least 30 minutes. Occlusion at either anastomosis during this period is of serious prognostic significance. Any anastomosis that is less than perfect should be resected and a fresh anastomosis of the affected vessels performed. All other alternatives carry a high risk of re-thrombosis with total loss of the testis.

Testicular biopsy (Fig. 12.10)
The tunica albuginea is incised away from the hilum and a sliver of tissue removed for biopsy. Arterial bleeding from the cut surface is a reassuring sign. Haemostasis is ensured and the biopsy site sutured with 6/0 Dexon.

The groin incision is closed in layers, carefully reconstructing the inguinal canal. Groin skin and scrotal incisions are sutured subcuticularly with fine absorbable material.

POSTOPERATIVE MONITORING AND CARE

Pulsation over the testicle can be easily detected with the Doppler probe. However, the procedure is disturbing to the child and unnecessary since late anastomotic occlusion in vessels which have remained patent for over 30 minutes at the time of operation is unusual. No additional measures beyond routine care for an extended orchidopexy are required. The child is mobilized and allowed home when comfortable within 24–72 hours.

CLINICAL SERIES

Several reports have appeared in the literature on the use of microsurgery in the treatment of undescended testes (Silber & Kelly 1976, Janecka & Romas 1979, MacMahon et al 1980, McC O'Brien et al 1983).

At the Royal Manchester Children's Hospital, a series (part reported by Bianchi 1984) of 35 testes in 29 children aged 3—15 years have been transferred to the scrotum by microvascular re-vascularization. Two testes were lost from failed arterial anastomoses and a second underwent late atrophy despite patent anastomoses. Seven children underwent bilateral procedures and one child had a single intra-abdominal testis. Operating time varied between 2.5 hours and 7 hours, with an average of 3.5 hours. Testicular ischaemia time varied from 1 to 2 hours. There was no postoperative morbidity or mortality and the children were allowed home within 2—4 days. One child has gone through puberty and has demonstrated definite growth in the transferred testis.

CONCLUSION

Microvascular orchidopexy is a safe and reliable technique for transfer of high undescended and intra-abdominal testes to the scrotum with a full blood supply. In these days of 'free flap' reconstruction and organ transplantation, e.g. of the liver, heart and kidney, anything less than a full blood supply to the transplanted tissue would be considered unacceptable. Equal standards should apply to the testis. It follows, therefore, that techniques which provide less than a full blood supply to the transferred testis should no longer be advocated.

The advantages or otherwise of orchidopexy for the high inguinal and intra-abdominal testis require long-term evaluation. Surgery should be performed before the end of the second year of life. Follow-up must encompass puberty and adulthood, with particular emphasis on fertility and malignancy in such transferred organs.

REFERENCES

Bianchi A 1984 Microvascular orchidopexy for high undescended testes. British Journal of Urology 56: 521—524

Corkery J J 1975 Staged orchidopexy—a new technique. Journal of Pediatric Surgery 10: 515—518

Fowler R, Stephens F D 1959 The role of testicular vascular anatomy in salvage of high undescended testes. Australian and New Zealand Journal of Surgery 29: 92—106

Hadziselimovic F 1977 Cryptorchidism: ultrastructure of normal and cryptorchid testis development. Advances in Anatomy, Embryology and Cell Biology 53: 3—71

Hausfeld K F, Schrandt D 1965 Malignancy of the testis following atrophy: report of three cases. Journal of Urology 94: 69—72

Hedinger C H R 1979 Histological data in cryptorchidism. Cryptorchidism, diagnosis and treatment. Pediatric and Adolescent Endocrinology 6: 3—13

Jackson M B, Chilvers C, Pike M C, Amsell P, Bull D 1986 Cryptorchidism: an apparent substantial increase since 1960. British Medical Journal 293: 1401—1404

Janecka I P, Romas N A 1979 Microvascular free transfer of human testes. Plastic and Reconstructive Surgery 63: 42—43

Levitt S B, Kogan S J, Engel R H, Weiss R M, Martin D C, Ehrlich R M 1978 The impalpable testis: a rational approach to management. Journal of Urology 120: 515—520

Ludwig G, Potempa J 1975 Der optimale zeitpunkt der behandlung des kryptorchismus. Deutsche Medizinische Wochenschrift 100: 680—683

McC O'Brien B, Rao V K, MacLeod A M, Morrison W A, MacMahon R A 1983 Microvascular testicular transfer. Plastic and Reconstructive Surgery 71: 87—90

MacMahon R A, Mc O'Brien B, Aberdeen J, Richardson W, Cussen L J 1980 Results of the use of autotransplantation of the intra-abdominal testis using microsurgical vascular anastomosis. Journal of Pediatric Surgery 15: 92—96

Martin D C, Menck H R 1975 The undescended testis: management after puberty. Journal of Urology 114: 77—79

Mengel W, Zimmerman F A, Hecker W C H 1981 Timing of repair for undescended testis. Yearbook Medical Publishers, Chicago, p 170

Scorer C G 1964 The descent of the testis. Archives of Disease in Childhood 39: 605—609

Silber S J, Kelly J 1976 Successful auto-transplantation of an intra-abdominal testis to the scrotum by microvascular techniques. Journal of Urology 115: 452—454

Chapter 13

Genitoplasty for virilizing congenital adrenal hyperplasia

Robert H. Whitaker

Introduction

The most common biochemical anomaly that leads to congenital adrenal hyperplasia is 21-hydroxylase deficiency. It is inherited as a recessive disorder and in approximately half the patients there is an associated salt loss. There is excessive conversion of 17-alpha-hydroxyprogesterone to weak adrenal androgens which in turn cause the virilization. All these female pseudohermaphrodites have a normal 46XX karyotype and normal development of ovaries, uterus and upper vagina.

ANATOMY

The degree of virilization is variable and can be mild with little more than an enlarged clitoris and fused labial folds (Fig. 13.1). In the severe forms the appearances are almost those of a normal cryptorchid male. In the mild form the vagina extends down to the urogenital sinus and is easily accessible surgically.

In the severe forms there is an upper vagina that connects to the posterior urethra via a small slit-like orifice (Fig. 13.2); surgical access is difficult. Most children show an intermediate degree of virilization between these two extremes.

INDICATIONS FOR SURGERY

As these children are otherwise normal females, and some will eventually become pregnant, it is important to correct the appearances of the external genitalia as perfectly as possible.

There are social and psychological advantages in correcting the anomaly early, perhaps before the age of 1 year, but technically the operation is easier when the child is older. Unless there are undue pressures for early correction, we tend to operate when the children are between 18 months and 2 years.

PREOPERATIVE PREPARATION

The diagnosis is confirmed by showing a normal female karyotype and abnormal plasma steroids. Laparotomy should not be needed to confirm the internal genital organs; an ultrasound scan can usually give all the information that is required. Radiographic studies after injection of contrast into the single opening show the details of the anatomy, but such a study may fail to show the vagina in a severely virilized child. Endoscopy is useful before commencing the reconstruction; it shows clearly the level of the confluence of the vagina and urethra and may be essential to show the slit-like vaginal opening in the posterior urethra.

The child should be biochemically stable before, and throughout, the operative and postoperative periods. Extra parenteral hydrocortisone is needed. If salt-losing, the dose of mineralocorticoids should be adjusted as necessary. Salt loss and blood pressure should be monitored carefully.

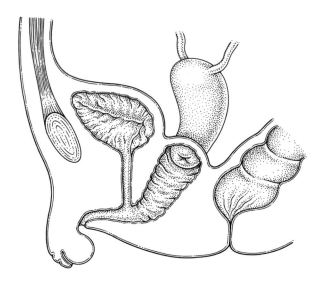

Fig. 13.1

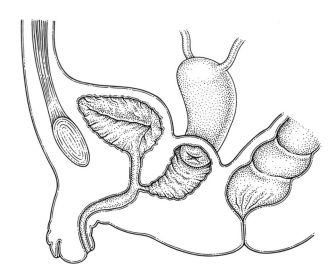

Fig. 13.2

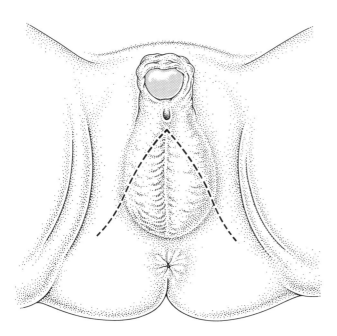

Fig. 13.3

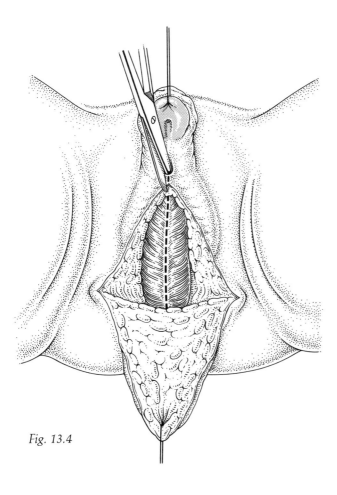

Fig. 13.4

SURGICAL TECHNIQUE

The operation reduces the phallus to a near normal sized clitoris; it exposes the urethra and opens the vagina to the perineum.

The skin is prepared and the child draped in the lithotomy position. If the virilization is minimal, all that is needed is a cut-back of the fused labia and a reduction of the clitoris as described below. The urethra and lower vagina are thus exposed. The urethra may be in a normal position but is usually a little hypospadiac.

Vaginoplasty

In severer forms of virilization a more extensive operation is necessary. The initial incision is a posteriorly based skin flap with the anterior tip just short of the common opening (Fig. 13.3). The flap is reflected posteriorly with its underlying fatty tissue.

The sinus is then opened from the common opening backwards until the urethra is seen, again usually in a hypospadiac position (Fig. 13.4).

The incision is extended beyond the urethra into the vagina and along its posterior midline until the widest point is reached (Fig. 13.5). The tip of the posteriorly based flap is then sutured into this vaginal incision and laterally around the lower edges of the vagina. As the suture line is extended down towards the perineum, the flap of skin becomes both the posterior wall of the vagina and also the posterior fourchette. 4/0 Dexon is used throughout.

In the most severely virilized children the vagina may enter the urethra high up in the urogenital sinus close to the bladder neck. An inlay vaginoplasty under these circumstances is difficult and will leave the patient with a severe female hypospadias. The level at which the vagina enters the urethra may well have been defined by the initial urethrogram. If this fails to demonstrate the vagina, endoscopy will reveal the site of the vaginal opening. Using an 8F cystoscope the vaginal opening is visualized and a Fogarty catheter is passed beside the cystoscope down the urogenital sinus and into the vagina (Fig. 13.6). The balloon is then inflated and the catheter occluded using a soft clamp.

The posterior skin flap is fashioned as for an inlay vaginoplasty. The urogenital sinus is cut back for a short way so as to position the external urinary meatus in a normal position.

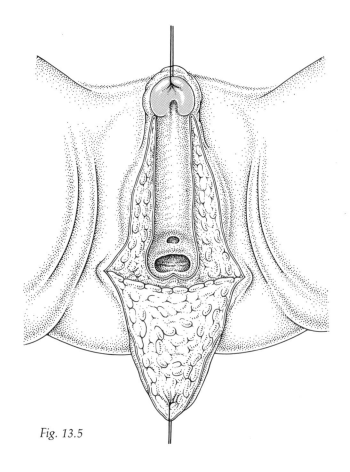

Fig. 13.5

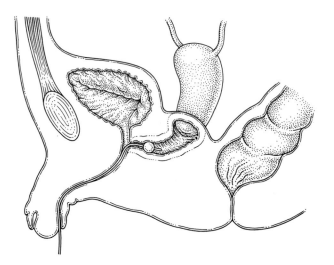

Fig. 13.6

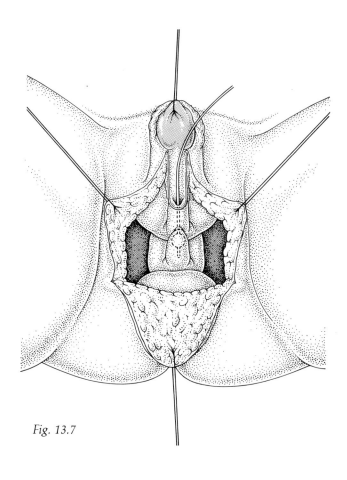

Fig. 13.7

The vagina is approached from below using palpation of the Fogarty balloon to help find the position of the vagina (Fig. 13.7).

The vagina is incised over the Fogarty balloon (Fig. 13.7). The balloon normally bursts at this point. Stay sutures are placed in the anterior vagina wall. The Fogarty catheter is removed and the posterior vaginal wall is separated from the proximal urethra using sharp dissection. This is a difficult part of the dissection because there is no easy plane between the vagina and the urethra at this point.

A size 10 Foley catheter is inserted down the urogenital sinus into the bladder. The opening in the posterior wall of what is now the neo-urethra is closed with two layers of interrupted 6/0 Dexon sutures (Fig. 13.8).

The posterior skin flap is sutured to the mobilized vagina (Figs 13.8, 13.9). No drain is necessary. A small pack using tulle-gras is placed within the vagina. Pressure dressing is then applied to the perineum using cross strapping.

The dressings are removed at 3 days with the child sedated. The catheter is removed at 4 days. Routine vaginal dilatation is wise, but if a good skin/vaginal anastomosis has been obtained this may be unnecessary.

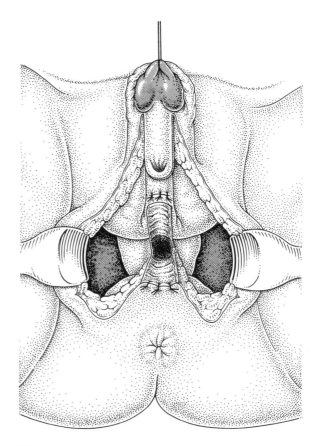

Fig. 13.8

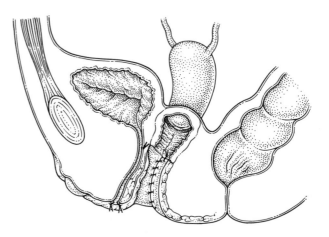

Fig. 13.9

Clitoral reduction

A stay suture is placed through the tip of the glans in preparation for the phallic reduction. The glans is preserved together with the ventral strip of opened corpus spongiosum which provides much of its blood supply. The dorsal neurovascular bundle is also preserved. A circumferential incision is made around the glans, retaining at least 1 cm of mucosa but leaving the ventral strip intact. The corpora cavernosa are exposed by dissecting the phallic skin downwards, and attention is turned to the dorsal aspect to isolate the dorsal neurovascular bundle. This is freed from the corpora, taking a strip of tunica if necessary to keep it intact. The dissection is stopped 1 cm from the glans where there are lateral ramifications of the nerve which must be preserved.

The ventral strip of corpus spongiosum is then dissected off the corpora cavernosa as far forwards as its attachment to the glans (Fig. 13.10). The corpora are cross-clamped and divided approximately 1 cm below the glans. The glans is thus attached by only the ventral mucosal strip and the dorsal neurovascular bundle. The corpora are dissected to their division and beyond towards their attachment to the bone. They are then transfixed, divided and excised.

The glans is fixed by suturing the cut edge of the corpora to the fibrous tissue over the periosteum of the undersurface of the pubic arch with 2 or 3 Dexon sutures. The site is adjusted so that the ventral mucosal strip lies neatly and the dorsal neurovascular bundle coils up under the pubic arch. The skin of the phallus is then unravelled and held up so that its blood supply can be inspected prior to midline incision. The mucosa that was left around the glans is now sewn to the deep edge of this incision and the two strips of phallic skin are brought backwards to form the two labia minora. Their medial edges are sutured to the lateral edges of the mucosal strip with continuous running 5/0 or 6/0 chromic catgut and their lateral edges to the rugose skin that represents the labia majora (Fig. 13.11a). Particular attention should be paid to the edges of the mucosal strip as haemorrhage can be a problem if it is not completely oversewn.

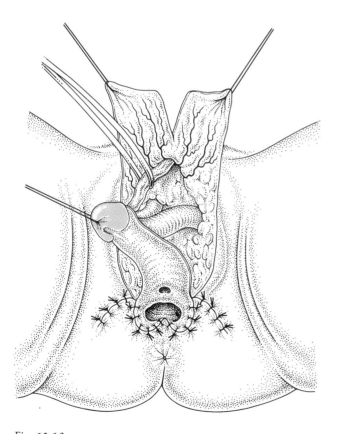

Fig. 13.10

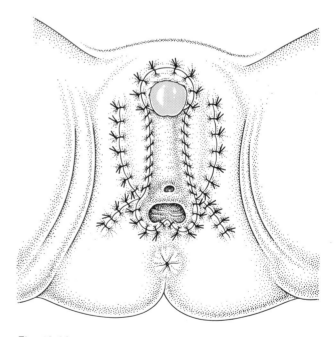

Fig. 13.11a

The posterior limit of the labia minora in most children is the junction with the posteriorly based skin flap, but for those in whom the sinus has been used for the lower urethra and in whom the anterior vaginal wall is bare, these posterior parts of the labia minora (phallic skin) can be extended up onto the anterior vaginal wall for a short distance, behind the urethra. 4/0 or 5/0 chromic catgut or Dexon can be used to close the skin. A small drain can be left in each posterior end of the wounds for 48 hours.

Figure 13.11a illustrates the end result of the procedure in low confluence of urethra and vagina whilst Figure 13.11b shows it in high confluence of urethra and vagina.

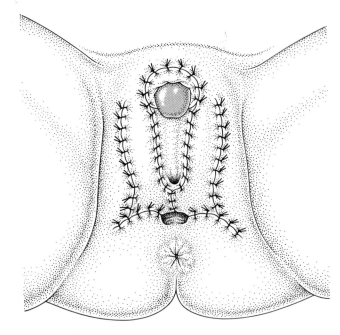

Fig. 13.11(b)

POSTOPERATIVE CARE

A urethral catheter is left in for 3—4 days. The vagina is packed with vaseline gauze which is removed after 48 hours. Vaginal dilatation is begun twice daily with a 1 cm diameter plastic dilator as soon as the pack is removed, and continued for at least a month or until such time as there is complete healing.

FOLLOW-UP

The child is seen regularly in outpatients until the wound is completely healed and then at yearly intervals until puberty. At that time an examination under anaesthetic is necessary to assess the adequacy of the vagina and the size of the clitoris. The clitoris may have appeared a little large at a younger age but at puberty it often seems more compatible with the general size of the child. If, at this stage, the clitoris seems too big, it can be reduced by excising its lateral aspects, but in our experience this has rarely been necessary. Any narrowing of the vagina can be corrected by swinging in flaps of nearby skin.

Chapter 14

Persistent Cloaca

Alberto Pena

Introduction

With this anomaly, which is encountered only in the female, there is an orifice on the perineum leading to a mucosal-lined channel into which the urinary, genital and alimentary systems terminate.

EMBRYOLOGY

The cloaca is a normal stage in embryogenesis, recognizable at the fifth week. Distally it opens into the tailgut, while proximally are the openings of the hindgut and the allantois. It is separated from the exterior of the embryo by the cloacal membrane. On either side of the cloaca, folds of mesoderm arise which fuse with each other from above downwards to form the urorectal septum. By the seventh week the cloaca is thus divided into the rectum posteriorly and the urogenital sinus anteriorly, and the cloacal membrane is divided into the urogenital and anal membranes.

Persistent cloaca is presumed to be due to arrest of formation of the urorectal septum; when the unstable cloacal membrane dehisces, the primitive cloaca then opens on the exterior. The relevant embryology is discussed by Pohlman (1911) and by Gray & Skandalakis (1972).

HISTORY AND INCIDENCE

The earliest mentions of patients with persistent cloaca in the English literature are those of Nordenfelt (1926) and Major (1929). They described patients who died shortly after they were born. Pennock & Stark (1926) published a paper entitled 'Persistence of Cloaca'; however, what they described was two patients with imperforate anus and recto-urethral fistula.

Interestingly, in large series of anorectal malformations such as the 162 cases of Ladd & Gross (1934), the 62 cases of Santulli (1952) and the 147 cases of Trusler & Wilkinson (1962), there was no mention of persistent cloaca. Table 14.1 summarizes the comparative frequency of persistent cloaca. We can roughly say that between 1 and 3.4% of anorectal malformations in females are

Table 14.1   Comparative frequency of persistent cloaca

	Anorectal malformations	Persistent cloaca	%
Both sexes			
Louw et al (1971)	287	6	2
Stephens & Smith (1971)	260	8	3
Nixon & Puri (1977)	86	1	1.1
Pena	370	47	12.7
Santulli et al (1971)	1166	23	1.9
Stephens & Smith (1971)	1098	27	2.4
Total	3276	112	3.4
Females			
Pena	143	47	32.8
Snyder (1966)	42	5	11.9
Palken et al (1972)	88	10	11.3
Bill et al (1975)	46	8	17.3
Total	319	70	21.9

persistent cloacas, and that 10–20% of all female anomalies correspond to this malformation. A careful chronological analysis of the numbers in the different series allows one to assume that the real frequency may be a little higher and may depend on the index of suspicion. On the other hand, the present author's frequency only reflects the tertiary nature of his institution and cannot be taken as representative of the real incidence of this defect since it receives a large number of referrals of complex anomalies from other hospitals.

ANATOMY, CLINICAL FINDINGS AND DIAGNOSIS

Based on the present author's experience, persistent cloaca must be considered as a spectrum of malformations with a common denominator or pattern consisting of the presence of one functioning external opening through which urine, genital secretions and faeces may be passed (Fig. 14.1). The understanding of the concept of spectrum will prove particularly useful when discussing treatment of the malformation (Fig. 14.2).

Although at first glance the external appearance of all these girls may be very similar (Fig. 14.1a), the real internal anatomy as seen through a panendoscope, or when widely exposed with a posterior sagittal operative approach, significantly varies from one case to another (Fig. 14.2). One important clinical clue to suspect the diagnosis is the presence of rather small looking genitalia in a girl with imperforate anus. The importance of an early suspicion cannot be over-emphasized, since the lack of correct diagnosis may induce the surgeon to believe that he is dealing with a case of a girl with a simple type of imperforate anus with vaginal fistula; he may subsequently repair the rectal component of the malformation only. The consequence of this is a girl with a pulled-through rectum and a persistent genitourinary sinus, the repair of which will be more difficult than the primary reconstruction which includes the repair both of the rectum and of the genitourinary tract. As can be seen in Fig. 14.2, the single channel or persistent cloaca communicates with rectum, vagina and urethra at different levels. The vagina is septate or double in 44% of cases in the author's experience (14.2f); this fact must be kept in mind by the surgeon when interpreting the radiological or endoscopic findings.

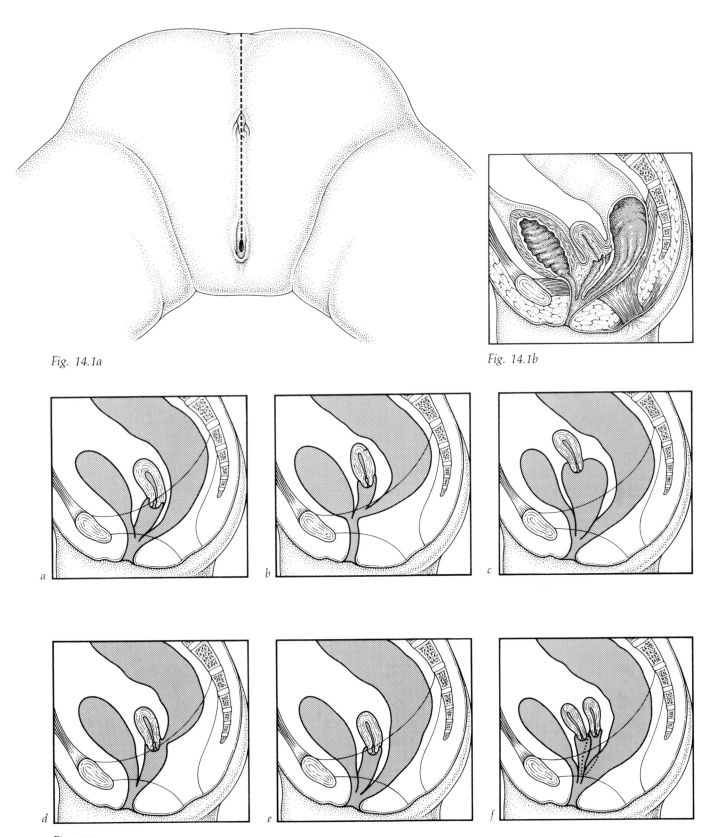

Fig. 14.1a

Fig. 14.1b

a

b

c

d

e

f

Fig. 14.2

Contrast X-ray studies must always include good lateral films to identify the three visceral components of the cloaca (Fig. 14.3). Precise interpretation is frequently difficult. However, since the advent of the posterior sagittal approach it is not so important to determine the precise and minute detail of the local anatomy since the approach to repair it will be initially the same. The combination of panendoscopy plus a 'cloacogram' (injection of contrast material through the single perineal hole) has proved useful enough to determine the basic characteristics of most cloacas. This can be complemented by contrast injection through the distal stoma of the colostomy when this is necessary. There is, however, a much more important evaluation to be done initially and this is the urological investigation, since these patients usually suffer from severe urological disturbances; in fact, genitourinary defects will account for most deaths. Studies may reveal renal agenesis, severe vesico-ureteric reflux or pelvi-ureteric obstruction. When severe sacral anomalies are present, one must also expect to deal with a neurogenic bladder.

It is common to find an associated hydrometrocolpos (Fig. 14.2c); in fact, when a cloaca is diagnosed or suspected in a patient with a lower abdominal mass, the surgeon can assume that an obstructed vagina is part of the malformation. The presence of a dilated vagina has been considered a cause of urinary obstruction and secondary infection (Cook & Marshall 1964). Also, sometimes these patients seem to empty their bladder into the genital tract, contributing to infection. It is debatable whether or not the distended vagina may provoke urinary obstruction, but the fact is that these babies may significantly improve after a vaginal decompression. Occasionally, in cases of double vagina, one may find the rectum

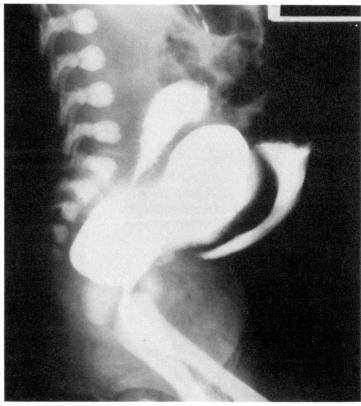

Fig. 14.3

opening between the vaginas. A significant size discrepancy between vaginas may also exist.

Rare types of cloaca include complex defects. The rectum may be located behind the urinary tract and open between the urinary tract and the vagina; the ureters may open ectopically, most frequently into the vagina.

Even more complex defects may include a large, wide cloaca, communicating with the intestine and ureter and without any recognizable bladder, vagina or rectum.

Important prognostic factors are: (a) the length of the common channel (cloaca), (b) the size of the vagina, (c) the condition of the sacrum, and (d) the quality of the muscles.

The common cloacal channel varies in length between 1 and 7 cm (Fig. 14.2a, b). It has been the present author's experience that those cases with a cloaca length of more than 3 cm cause technical difficulty in mobilizing the vagina down to reach the labia. The surgeon is then obligated to try some other technical alternative to fill the gap between vagina and perineum, as will be discussed later. Common channels of less than 3 cm usually allow a primary suture between vagina and perineum. The size of the vagina is also relevant. A small vagina is more difficult to dissect and mobilize; it is also more likely to become devascularized. A large vagina allows the surgeon an easier mobilization and also the possibility of using a flap from its dome to fill the gap in cases of long common channel (Kimura et al 1985).

A complete sacrum usually indicates that the pelvic innervation is normal and, therefore, the prognosis in terms of bowel and urinary continence is good. One sacral vertebra missing does not seem to have any adverse effect on faecal and urinary continence.

The quality of the sphincter muscles can usually be predicted by looking at the patient's perineum. A marked midline groove and a distinct recognizable anal dimple are usually associated with a good external anal sphincter and levator muscle.

TREATMENT

Establishing therapeutic priorities when dealing with a newborn with this malformation is the key to avoiding neonatal deaths. One must remember that there are two real emergencies requiring urgent treatment and these are intestinal obstruction and the urinary problem. Therefore a urological evaluation is mandatory and must be done even before the colostomy is performed, particularly if the baby is showing signs of sepsis. Thus, the surgeon will be in the position to plan a procedure to decompress the colon and the urinary or genital tract simultaneously.

Before 1953 there were, in the English literature, isolated reports of cloacal deformities, but the babies were either born dead or else died shortly after birth.

In 1958, Sieber & Klein reported two cases; one died and the other was referred to Orvar Swenson who performed the first simultaneous urethral, vaginal and rectal reconstruction in 1953.

Gough (1959) reviewed 18 cases from the Great Ormond Street experience; 11 patients died. Therapeutic attempts included colostomies, urinary diversion and abdomino-perineal pull-through for the rectal part of the defect. No mention was made concerning the management of the genitourinary sinus.

Bock & Madsen (1971) published a case report. The patient underwent an abdomino-perineal pull-through for the rectum only and the genitourinary sinus was left untouched.

In 1973, Raffensperger & Ramenofsky, on the basis of their experience with 15 patients treated in different ways, proposed that the urinary, genital and gastrointestinal tracts must all be separated from one another in the newborn period. Two of their patients received a vaginal abdomino-perineal pull-through in the newborn period. This paper represents the first series illustrating the multiple complications that must be expected when dealing with persistent cloacas.

Cheng et al (1974) published their experience with five cases, two of which died. They recommended a multiple-stage approach, including a colostomy during the newborn period, followed by a rectal pull-through between the ages of 10 and 15 months and a genitoplasty later in life. This paper includes a good literature review of 50 cases previously published, emphasizing the high incidence of associated anomalies of the genital (77%) and urinary (63%) systems.

Kay & Tank (1977) published a review of five patients seen at their centre and 34 documented cases; they also emphasized the high frequency of co-existing anomalies of the urinary tract (33%) and other systems and organs. They proposed a right transverse colostomy in the newborn period followed by rectal and vaginal pull-through when the patient weighs 25 pounds in cases of high vaginal opening. In cases of low vaginal opening they prefer a vaginoplasty by a posterior flap to be done when the child is 10–12 years old.

Mollitt et al (1981) published an important paper pointing out the importance of long-term follow-up in these patients since they may suffer from obstructed vaginas or uteri with severe symptoms later in life.

Hendren (1977, 1980, 1982, 1986) published four papers which together represent the largest, most ambitious and knowledgeable personal experience ever published on the subject. By reading them one can see that the author has really been exposed to the spectrum of malformations; many of his cases were referred to him as secondary problems and therefore present additional and more complicated therapeutic challenges. His series demonstrates very well the magnitude of the effort required to treat these cases and that it must only be carried out by knowledgeable, experienced, meticulous and skilled paediatric surgeons, trained also in paediatric urology.

Skin flaps may be useful to allow suture of the vagina to the skin, and vaginal tubularization may be needed in cases of large vaginas (Kimura et al 1985). Bowel interposition may save some apparently 'non useful' vaginas (Harrison et al 1983).

Many of the previously proposed treatments may work for certain kinds of persistent cloacas but will not be useful for others. This can only be acknowledged by understanding the concept of the spectrum of this group of defects. Thus, a simple perineal approach could conceivably be enough to repair a simple low defect (Fig. 14.2e). This variant is unfortunately very unusual.

A posterior sagittal approach may be sufficient to repair most variants of this defect (Fig. 14.2a, b, e, f).

A posterior sagittal approach and laparotomy would be indicated for the repair of a high rectal opening, such as the one shown in Figure 14.2d, in order to allow one to mobilize the bowel.

The same approach would be necessary to repair a defect with a long common channel, such as the one shown in Figure 14.2b; in this case the justification for the laparotomy would be the long gap existing between vagina and perineum.

Different combinations of defects (other than those shown in Fig. 14.2a–f) must be expected.

Posterior sagittal ano-recto-vagino-urethroplasty

Since 1982 the present author (Pena 1982, 1985, 1986) has been treating persisting cloacas with a new ambitious operation repairing the rectal, vaginal and urethral components in a single procedure called posterior sagittal ano-recto-vagino-urethroplasty (PSARVUP). The basic steps when dealing with a new persistent cloaca case include:

a. Establishing therapeutic priorities in the newborn in order to treat the most pressing or life-threatening defect (usually urinary obstruction).
b. Performance of a completely diverting descending colostomy (double barrel). In addition, when necessary, vaginal and/or bladder decompression must be performed simultaneously.
c. PSARVUP on elective basis when the child is older than 6 months. The discussion will be limited to the repair of the cloaca itself, granted that the urinary problem must be treated on an individual basis before, during or after PSARVUP, depending on the circumstances.

The main object of the posterior sagittal operation is to attain, when feasible, in a single operation:

a. Faecal continence
b. Urinary continence
c. Normal sexual function

In the author's experience most cloacas can be successfully reconstructed with this procedure and only a minority will require a laparotomy, perineal skin flaps, vaginal flap or bowel interposition.

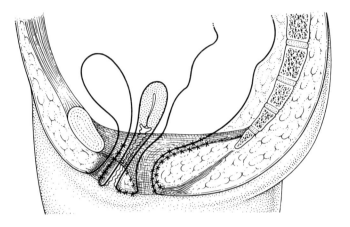

The operation consists of a posterior sagittal incision with full exposure of the entire malformation, separation of the three visceral components, and construction of a neo-urethra using the single cloacal channel, vaginal and rectal pull-throughs with preservation of the entire striated muscle mechanism (levator muscle complex and external sphincter) (Fig. 14.4a, b).

Fig. 14.4a

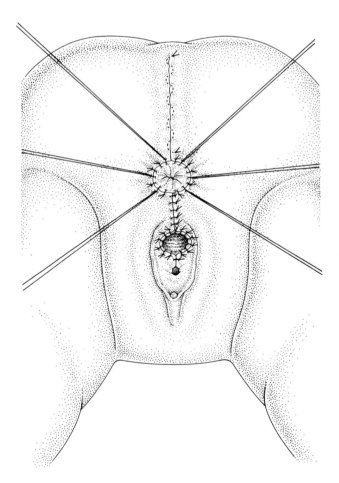

Fig. 14.4b

The patient is placed in a prone position with the pelvis elevated. No attempt is made to place a urinary catheter preoperatively, since it is difficult to direct it from outside. The incision runs from the mid-sacrum down to the cloacal orifice, dividing all the muscle structures behind the viscera (Fig. 14.5a). The external sphincter and muscle complex must be divided, including both their posterior and anterior aspects. The surgeon must remain strictly in the midline during the entire operation. To achieve this, a symmetrical contraction of the striated muscles on both sides of the midline when electrically stimulated must be appreciated, and also one must preserve a very fine midline sagittal fascia which will avoid herniation of fat into the operative field. Staying in the midline guarantees avoiding any neurological damage since all nerves run paramedially and are terminal at midline.

A needle-tip cautery is used through the entire operation and scrupulous haemostasis is essential to be able to recognize the important muscle and visceral structures. Deep to the skin, the longitudinal fibres of the external sphincter are identified. They run from the coccyx to the anal site. Deeper into the muscle, one will find more fat tissue, which separates the sphincter muscle fibres from the levator muscle at the cephalad part of the incision. For more information related to the anatomical and functional details of these muscles, the reader is referred to previous publications by the present author. Two sharp Weitlaner retractors provide excellent exposure but they must be placed superficially so as not to crush the muscles. The coccyx is split in the midline, a right-angle clamp is introduced through the split coccyx into the pre-sacral space, and the levator muscle is divided in the midline. After this, a visceral structure is found; its external appearance does not allow one to elucidate whether it is rectum, vagina or the cloacal channel (Fig. 14.5a). This structure must, therefore, be opened in the midline, holding its wall edges apart by 5/0 silk stitches (Fig. 14.5b). By looking inside, one may determine the precise anatomical variant with which one is dealing (Fig. 14.5c). It is at this point that one may predict whether a laparotomy, perineal skin flaps, labial or vaginal flap or else bowel interposition as a vaginal substitute will be required. In the author's experience, whenever the rectum is identified through this approach, a laparotomy will not be necessary since with an adequate technique the bowel can be pulled down to the skin without tension. If the rectum is not seen through this approach, a laparotomy will be required to bring it down.

The vagina usually presents a more difficult problem. High, small vaginas are the most challenging; large, low vaginas are easy to deal with and one can expect much better results from such cases.

Sometimes it is difficult to predict whether or not a laparotomy will be required for vaginal construction, even with the malformation exposed. One may have to start trying to dissect and mobilize the vagina, only to find after a while that a laparotomy is indeed needed since the vagina is too high to be pulled down.

Once the malformation is completely exposed (Fig. 14.5c), the goal is then to achieve separation of the three structures. It is important to remember that they actually share a common wall immediately above the point of union. A plane of dissection should be created between rectum and vagina and subsequently between vagina and urethra. This manoeuvre will consume most of the time employed in this repair (usually 4–9 hours). To avoid tissue damage, many 6/0 silk mucosal stitches are used for traction. The injection of 1:100 000 adrenaline solution allows an easier separation of the structures.

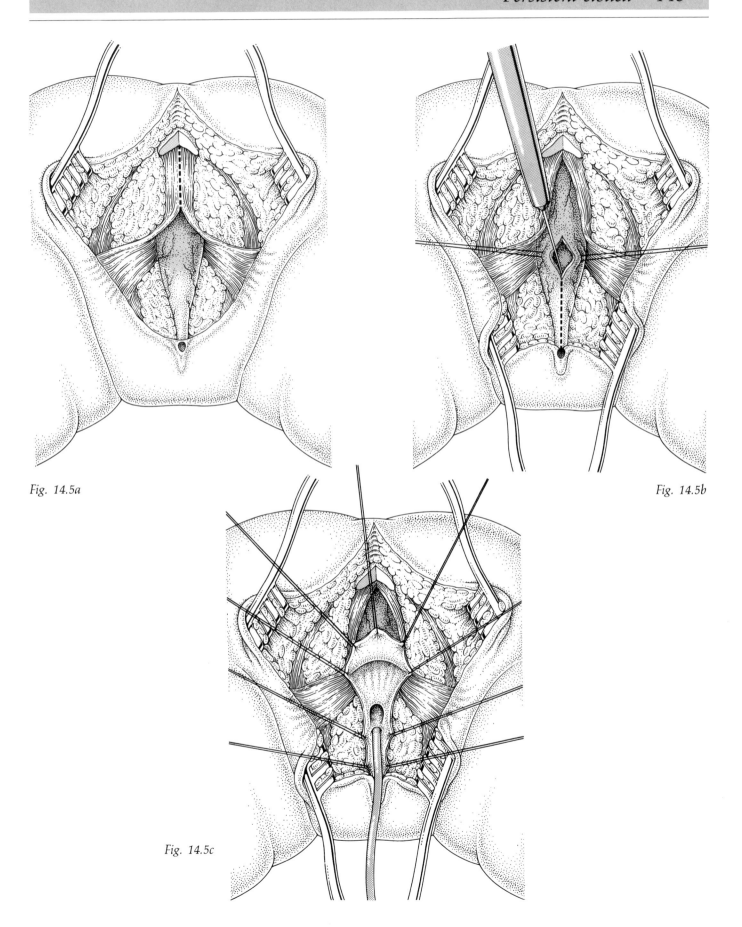

Fig. 14.5a

Fig. 14.5b

Fig. 14.5c

The rectum is separated from the vagina and mobilized enough to be sutured to the skin (Fig. 14.6a). The length of the common wall between rectum and vagina varies from one case to another; higher rectal openings have shorter common walls.

The separation of vagina from the urinary tract is a more difficult manoeuvre and requires more skill since both structures have friable tissue (Fig. 14.6b). It is convenient to remain closer to the vaginal lumen than to the urethral side in order to protect the urinary sphincter and avoid urinary fistulae. The neo-urethra must be constructed by using the common cloacal channel (Fig. 14.6c). This full exposure of the area and its correlation with the results obtained has allowed the present author to clarify an important anatomical misconception related to the urinary sphincter. This structure has been considered and depicted as a well-limited ring muscle band which must be protected to attain urinary continence. A meticulous dissection and search did not allow the author to identify any similar structure in cases that were subsequently demonstrated to be urinary continent. The urinary sphincter, therefore, seems to be represented in these cases by a continuum of striated muscle existing all along the common channel which will function as a neo-urethra. This muscle is easily identifiable by electrical stimulation. Urinary continence depends upon the preservation of this muscle as well as a good sacrum, and it is not predictable on the basis of endoscopic or radiological findings nor from the distance existing between the external opening and the rectal, urethral and vaginal orifices.

A vaginal septum, frequently found, can be easily resected during the operation.

A very large vagina may require tapering in order to create an introitus proportionate to the size of the girl's perineum.

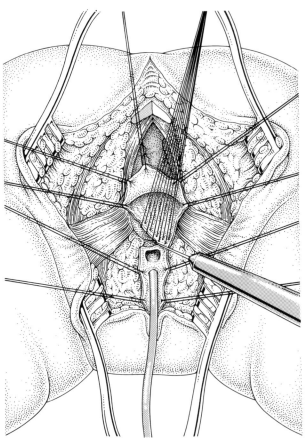

Fig. 14.6a

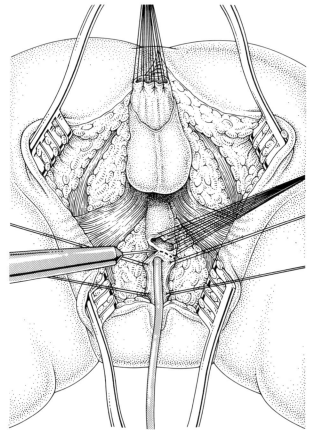

Fig. 14.6b

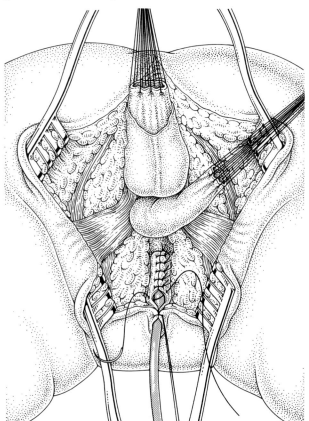

Fig. 14.6c

The vaginal wall is then sutured to the perineal skin using separate stitches of an absorbable synthetic material. The perineal body must be reconstructed; for this, the anterior and posterior limits of the external sphincter and muscle complex are determined using the electrical stimulator. The anterior limit of the muscle complex is re-approximated using interrupted 5/0 Vycril stitches (Fig. 14.7a). The rectum will be located in front of the levator muscles and within the limits of the muscle complex and external sphincter. The width of the rectum cannot be larger than the muscle complex width. In cases with a larger rectum it is imperative to tailor it to achieve our goal; this happens in more than 50% of cases. The amount of rectum resected depends on the size discrepancy.

The tapering is carried out, resecting part of the posterior rectal wall and closing with two layers of interrupted stitches. The sutures that bring together both posterior edges of the muscle complex must be anchored to the posterior rectal wall to avoid rectal prolapse (Fig. 14.7b).

The anoplasty is achieved with 16 stitches of interrupted 5/0 Vycril (Fig. 14.7c). A Foley catheter or a supra-pubic cystostomy tube is left in place for 10–14 days.

Anal dilatations are started 2 weeks after the operation. These are performed twice daily by the mother, and every week the surgeon must pass the next larger sized dilator. The goal is to reach a 12 Hegar dilator in newborns or young infants, a 15 Hegar in 1-year-old patients and a 16 or 17 Hegar in school-age children before considering closure of the colostomy. This process usually takes between 2 and 3 months. After the colostomy has been closed, the last-sized dilator must be passed daily and a gradual tapering in frequency can be carried out over a 6-month period.

We have not dilated the vagina postoperatively. The vaginal introitus of these girls frequently looks rather narrow, but endoscopic examination 3 months after surgery usually shows a very satisfactory vagina. A few of our patients have already reached puberty and we have observed that the oestrogen secretion enlarges the vagina even more.

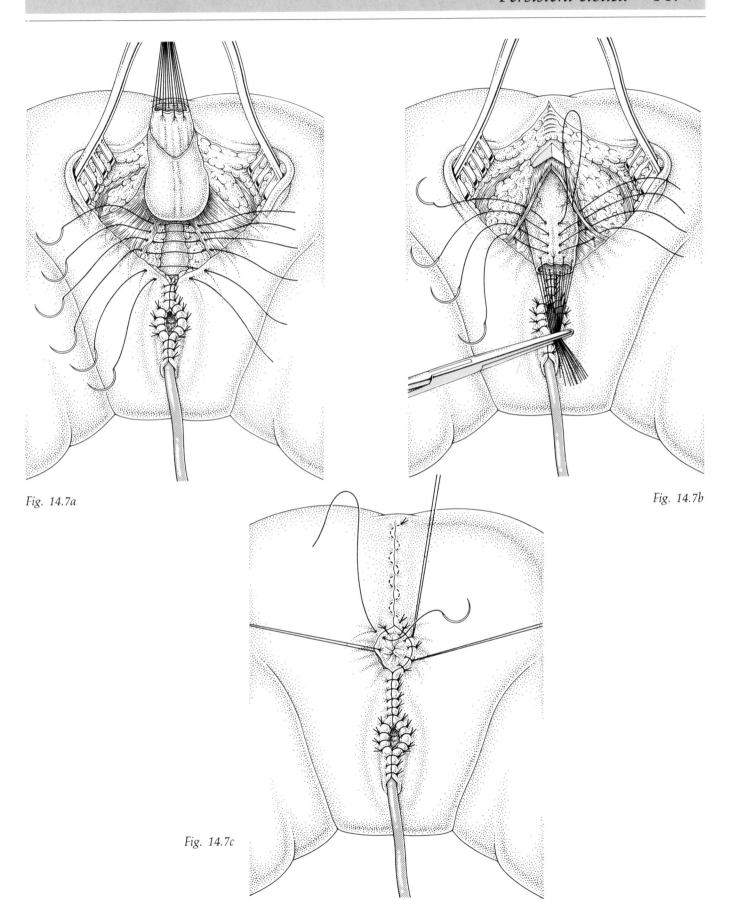

Fig. 14.7a

Fig. 14.7b

Fig. 14.7c

Re-operations for persistent genitourinary sinus

The most frequent indication for re-operation of persistent cloaca is a school-age or teenage patient who was born with this defect and was operated on with conventional techniques prior to the advent of PSARVUP. The most common way of treatment was by a rectal pull-through, leaving intact the genitourinary sinus. The patients may or may not have had good faecal and/or urinary control. Under these circumstances the treatment consists of creating a protective right transverse colostomy, followed by a secondary PSARVUP, and in a third stage the colostomy is closed.

The reason for recommending a right transverse colostomy rather than a descending one, as we do for primary cases, is related to the fact that most patients who previously underwent a pull-through procedure most likely had a ligation of the inferior mesenteric or left colic artery; the entire left colon is therefore supplied by the middle colic vessels and by the new blood supply formed between the perianal area and the rectum. Under these circumstances a descending colostomy may compromise the blood supply of the distal colon.

In these cases the rectum is usually found mislocated either too anteriorly or lateral to the muscle complex and external sphincter. Usually, the external sphincter and muscle complex are found intact. The operation consists of a full midline sagittal incision, dividing the external sphincter and muscle complex. Multiple 5/0 silk traction stitches are placed at the mucocutaneous junction of the anus. A meticulous dissection is carried out around the rectum, staying as close as possible to the bowel serosa and leaving intact all the striated muscle in the vicinity. For the identification of such muscle, we use the electrical stimulator. Once the rectum has been completely mobilized, the genitourinary sinus is exposed as in the second part of the original primary cloaca repair (Fig. 14.6b). We then proceed with the repair of the vagina and the urinary tract as was previously described. The perineal body is also repaired. Many of these patients had a previous abdomino-perineal operation and therefore they have colon pulled down to the perineum. To preserve the blood supply of the colon, the previous surgeon was obligated to mobilize a piece of mesentery with it, which subsequently leaves a bulging mass surrounding the colon, interfering with a good muscle–bowel contact and therefore being disadvantageous for bowel continence. In these cases we resect the mesentery that surrounds the rectum along the last few centimetres, leaving the blood supply of the bowel to its transmural vessels. So far, no cases of bowel ischaemia have been recorded in the author's experience. The rectum is then relocated anterior to the levator muscle, within the limits of the muscle complex and at the centre of the external sphincter.

Some patients who were previously apparently suffering from urinary incontinence obtained urinary control, and the explanation is that they were previously urinating into a large vagina and subsequently dribbling urine. Once we successfully separated the vagina from the urinary tract, the patient was able to urinate and have control. In other cases, with a poor sacrum and a primary neurogenic bladder, the separation of vagina from the urinary tract was also advantageous for the patient, since now she was able to intermittently catheterize the bladder because the new urethral orifice was easily visible. Patients with genitourinary sinus or persistent cloaca usually cannot practise intermittent catheterization.

In some cases of re-operation we find, as in primary cases, a long gap between vagina and perineum so that it is impossible to mobilize the vagina enough without risking its vascularization. In those cases, we may take advantage of the fact that many of these patients have colon with mesentery pulled down as a rectum and therefore we may elect to use the most distal part of this bowel, preserving its mesentery, to fill the gap between vagina and perineum. The bowel proximal is then mobilized, pulled down posterior to the vagina and anastomosed to the skin within the limits of the external sphincter. By doing this, we do not have to open the abdomen.

SECONDARY OPERATIONS FOR THE TREATMENT OF FAECAL AND URINARY INCONTINENCE

Patients with poor sacrums and demonstrated neurogenic bladders are not good candidates for re-operation using the posterior sagittal approach. On the other hand, patients with good sacrums, good-looking perineums, evidence of a large vagina, and urinary incontinence must be re-operated on because of the reasons discussed above.

Faecal incontinence in these patients may be the result of a mislocated rectum. The ideal candidate for a re-operation for the treatment of such incontinence is a patient with a good sacrum, good muscles and evidence of a completely mislocated rectum. The rectum most frequently is sited too anteriorly to the external sphincter and the muscles remain intact. In the author's experience, re-operation carried out in patients with poor sacrums renders rather poor results.

RESULTS

Forty-seven patients in the present author's series have undergone a posterior sagittal ano-recto-vagino-urethroplasty. Most are too young to be evaluated at the present time. However, we recently evaluated 23 patients older than 3 years of age and found that 18 had voluntary bowel movements, 17 suffered from occasional soiling in their underwear and 14 were urinary continent. Some of the patients who did not have voluntary bowel movements and suffered from urinary incontinence were still between 3 and 4 years old. Four patients had differing degrees of sacral abnormality.

Complications related to the procedure include one case in which the vagina retracted and sloughed because of de-vascularization during the dissection. Three patients suffered from urethro-vaginal fistula and are still waiting for a solution to that problem. There have been no wound infections and no bowel–skin anastomosis dehiscence. The vagina in all patients looked well endoscopically 3 months after the procedure, although in some, the external introitus was rather narrow.

It was necessary to open the abdomen to complete the repair in seven cases. Labial skin flaps were used to fill the gap between vagina and perineum in 10 patients. A bowel interposition for vaginal replacement was used in two cases, and in two more cases the distal vagina was reconstructed using a flap from its own dome.

REFERENCES

Bill A H, Hall D G, Johnson R J 1975 Position of rectal fistula in relation to the hymen in 46 girls with imperforate anus. Journal of Pediatric Surgery 10: 361–365

Bock J E, Madsen C M 1971 Anorectal atresia with rectocloacal fistula. Acta Chirurgica Scandinavica 137: 284–286

Cheng G K, Fisher J H, O'Hare K H, Retik A B, Darling D B 1974 Anomaly of the persistent cloaca in female infants. American Journal of Roentgenology 120: 413–423

Cook G T, Marshall V F 1964 Hydrocolpos causing urinary obstruction. Journal of Urology 92: 127–132

Gough M H 1959 Anorectal agenesis with persistence of cloaca. Proceedings of the Royal Society of Medicine 52: 886–889

Gray S W, Skandalakis J E 1972 The colon and rectum. In: Embryology for surgeons. W B Saunders, Philadelphia, chap. 6, p 187–216

Harrison M R, Glick P L, Nakayama D K, de Lorimier A A 1983 Loop colon rectovaginoplasty for high cloacal anomaly. Journal of Pediatric Surgery 18: 885–886

Hendren W H 1977 Surgical management of urogenital sinus abnormalities. Journal of Pediatric Surgery 12: 339–357

Hendren W H 1980 Urogenital sinus and anorectal malformation: experience with 22 cases. Journal of Pediatric Surgery 15: 628–641

Hendren W H 1982 Further experience in reconstructive surgery for cloacal anomalies. Journal of Pediatric Surgery 17: 695–717

Hendren W H 1986 Repair of cloacal anomalies: current techniques. Journal of Pediatric Surgery 21: 1159–1176

Johnson R J, Palken M. Derrick W, Bill A H 1972 The embryology of high anorectal and associated genitourinary anomalies in the female. Surgery, Gynecology and Obstetrics 135: 759–762

Kay R, Tank E S 1977 Principles of management of the persistent cloaca in the female newborn. Journal of Urology 117: 102–104

Kimura K, Ueoka K, Tsugawach, Tanikaze S, Matsumoto Y 1985 Reconstructive surgery for cloacal anomalies. Zeitschrift fur Kinderchirurgie 40: 31–35

Ladd W E, Gross R E 1934 Congenital malformations of anus and rectum. Report of 162 cases. American Journal of Surgery 23: 167–183

Louw J H, Cywes S, Cremin B J 1971 The management of anorectal agenesis. South African Journal of Surgery 9: 21–30

Major S G 1929 Persistence of the cloaca: report of case. Minnesota Medicine 12: 96–97

Mollitt D L, Schullinger J N, Santulli T V, Hensle T W 1981 Complications at menarche of urogenital sinus with associated anorectal malformations. Journal of Pediatric Surgery 16: 349–352

Nixon H H, Puri P 1977 The results of treatment of anorectal anomalies: a thirteen to twenty year follow up. Journal of Pediatric Surgery 12: 27–37

Nordenfelt O 1926 Two cases of cloacal formation with congenital hydrometra and hydrocolpos. Acta Gynecologica 5: 1–23

Palken M, Johnson R J, Derrick W, Bill A H 1972 Clinical aspects of female patients with high anorectal agenesis. Surgery, Gynecology and Obstetrics 135: 411–416

Pena A 1985 Surgical treatment of high imperforate anus. World Journal of Surgery 9: 236–243

Pena A 1986 Posterior sagittal approach for the correction of anorectal malformations. Advances in Surgery 19: 69–100

Pena A, DeVries P 1982 Posterior sagittal anorectoplasty: important technical considerations and new applications. Journal of Pediatric Surgery 17: 796–811

Pennock W J, Stark W J 1926 Persistence of cloaca. Journal of Urology 16: 93–95

Pohlman A G 1911 The development of the cloaca in human embryos. American Journal of Anatomy 12: 1–26

Raffensperger J G, Ramenofsky M L 1973 The management of a cloaca. Journal of Pediatric Surgery 8: 647–657

Santulli T V 1952 The treatment of imperforate anus and associated fistulas. Surgery, Gynecology and Obstetrics 95: 601–614

Santulli T V, Schullinger J N, Kieseweter W B, Bill A H 1971 Imperforate anus: a survey from the members of the Surgical Section of the American Academy of Pediatrics. Journal of Pediatric Surgery 6: 484–487

Sieber W K, Klein R 1958 Cloaca with non-adrenal female pseudohermaphroditism. Pediatrics 22: 472–477

Snyder W H 1966 Some unusual forms of imperforate anus in female infants. American Journal of Surgery 11: 319–325

Stephens F D, Smith E D 1971 Ano-rectal malformations in children. Year Book Medical Publishers, Chicago, chap. 7, p 160–171

Trusler G A, Wilkinson R H 1962 Imperforate anus: a review of 147 cases. Canadian Journal of Surgery 5: 269–277

Chapter 15

The surgery of bladder exstrophy and epispadias

Howard M. Snyder III

Newborn exstrophy closure

Babies born with bladder exstrophy should have the bladder closed within the first 48 hours of life unless there are medical contraindications to surgery. The presence of maternal relaxin makes the pelvic bones flexible and the pubis symphysis can be approximated without pelvic osteotomies. Careful peroperative monitoring of the baby and appropriate precautions to maintain a normal body temperature are essential, as this is a lengthy operation. A blood transfusion may be needed, especially in the male.

Circumferential prepping and draping of the baby from chest to calf is required, so that the assistant can grasp the thighs and approximate the symphysis in the later stages of the operation without contaminating the operative field.

THE OPERATION

Bilateral small ureteric stents are inserted. Two paraexstrophy skin flaps are raised (Fig. 15.1). They should be approximately 1 cm wide, and to achieve this width it may be necessary to make the incision laterally beyond the shiny paraexstrophy skin. The flaps are mobilized distally to allow exposure of the pubic bones. The incision across the urethral plate must be sufficiently distal to the veru to avoid the prostate. The umbilical cord is excised. In the female, paraexstrophy flaps are also raised with an incision dividing the urethral plate above the front wall of the vagina.

It is important when raising the para-exstrophy flaps to keep them thick with a broad base so as to preserve their blood supply. Distal mobilization is continued until the pubic bone is exposed (Fig. 15.2). Beneath the upper end of the flaps the perivesical extra-peritoneal space is then entered and mobilization of the bladder commenced. Dissection continues distally, following the medial edge of the rectus muscle until the pubic bone is reached. By staying close to the medial border of the symphysis, the inter-symphyseal band is delineated.

After freeing the symphyseal attachment of the intersymphyseal band from the pubic bone, the dissection continues distally along the corporal bodies (Fig. 15.3). The dorsal nerves lie laterally and are not usually seen in a neonatal repair. If the dissection is kept close to the corpora, the prostate can be mobilized with little bleeding. It must be completely mobilized with the bladder in order to release corporal tethering and allow the later placement of the bladder into the pelvis.

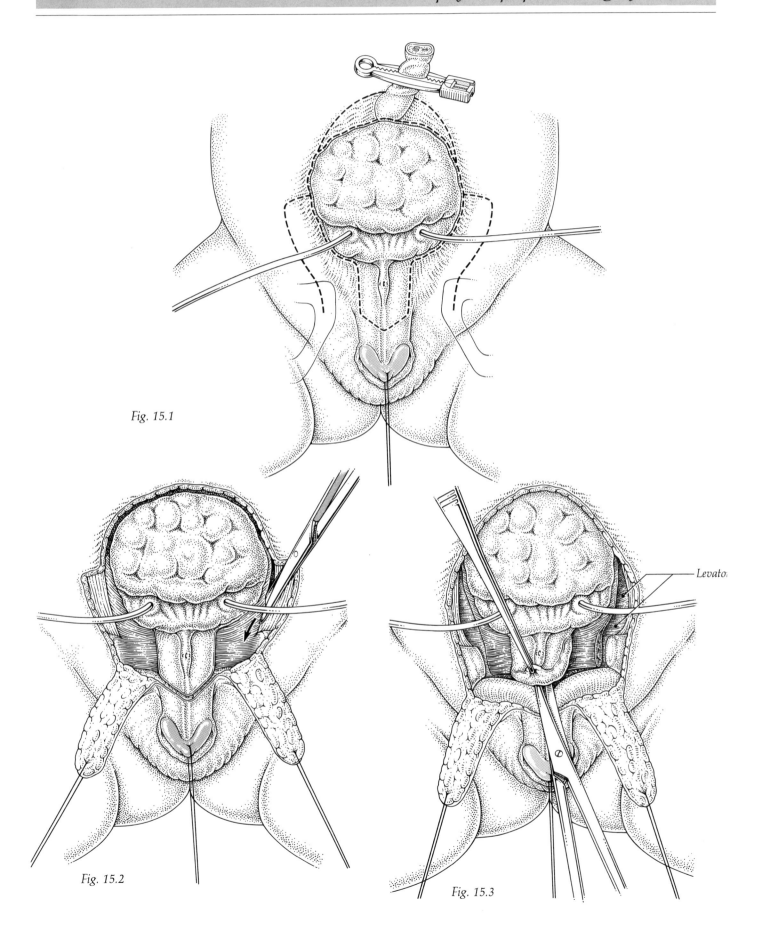

Fig. 15.1

Fig. 15.2

Fig. 15.3

Levato

The intersymphyseal band is mobilized off the levator muscle (male) or the front wall of the vagina (female) in order to allow reconstruction of the bladder neck without lateral tethering. There is a variable degree of tethering of the corpora to the pubic bones and this is released by dissecting close to the bone (Fig. 15.4a). A periosteal elevator is a useful instrument for this part of the dissection.

The mobilization of the corpora continues until the plane of the levator muscle is reached. As the deep vessels to the corpora travel in Alcock's canal, which is deep to the plane of the levator muscle, their blood supply is protected. Much of the release of the tethering of the corpora is achieved by adequate mobilization of the prostate gland. Freeing the corpora from the pubic bone (Fig. 15.4b) will not produce a good dependent angle unless the prostate has been completely freed.

Mobilization of the bladder continues using sharp dissection until it is free from the rectus fascia. The peritoneum is swept off the dome and body so that the closed bladder can be placed in the pelvis behind the peritoneum (Fig. 15.4c). The ureters are often seen during this part of the mobilization and must be protected.

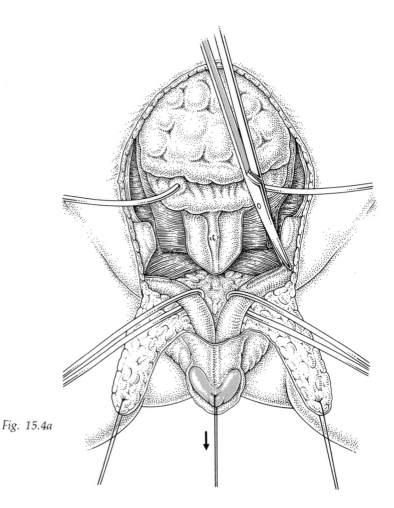

Fig. 15.4a

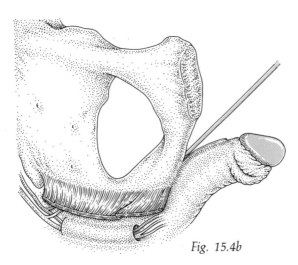

Fig. 15.4b

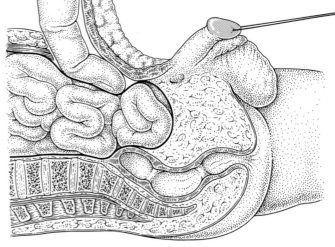

Fig. 15.4c

The paraexstrophy flaps are sutured together in the midline and to the mobilized urethral plate and bladder, so that when the rudimentary bladder neck is closed, an epithelial stricture is avoided (Fig. 15.5). The width of this epithelial strip should be approximately 2 cm. 5/0 and 6/0 polyglycolic acid (Dexon) or polyglactan (Vicryl) sutures are used.

The ureteric stents are brought out through the bladder wall and a size 10 or 12F Malecot suprapubic catheter is placed low on the back wall of the bladder just above the trigone (Fig. 15.6). If the bladder is small and the mucosa very hypertrophied and polypoid, bladder closure may be facilitated by excising the hypertrophic mucosa using diathermy. For very small bladders, stretching with or without superficial incision of the detrusor on its outer aspect may help to close the bladder. Closure is begun superiorly using a 3/0 Vicryl suture, picking up a small amount of mucosa with a larger bite of the muscle.

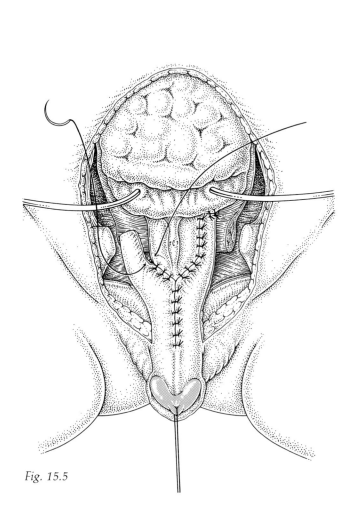

Fig. 15.5

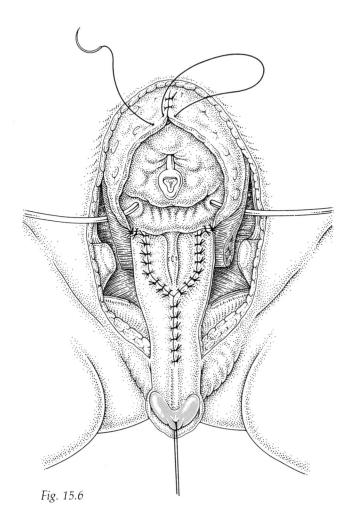

Fig. 15.6

The lateral edges of the paraexstrophy flaps are sutured together so as to create a urethra long enough to reach from the proposed pelvic position of the bladder to the anterior abdominal wall (Fig. 15.7). Interrupted sutures along these paraexstrophy flaps induce less ischaemia and allow the urethra to stretch more easily.

The bladder closure is continued with a second inverting layer of sutures (Fig. 15.8). As this closure progresses distally, it reconstructs the bladder neck by approximating the intersymphyseal band. If this band has been adequately mobilized, the bladder neck will not be tethered open and functional reconstruction of the bladder is then independent of the position of the pelvic bones.

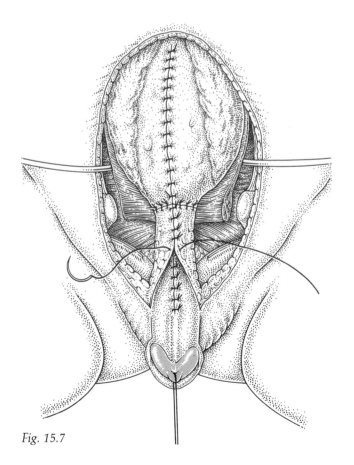

Fig. 15.7

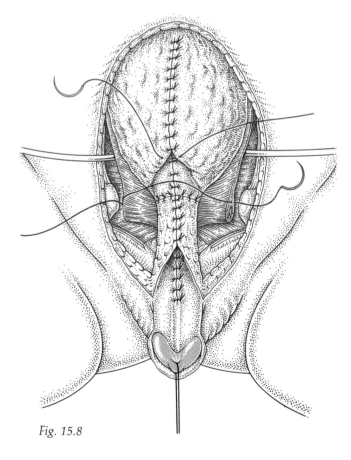

Fig. 15.8

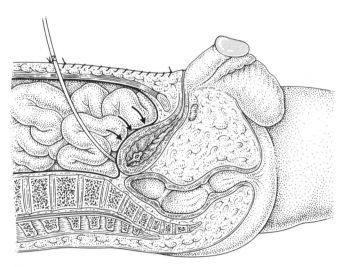

Fig. 15.9a

The closed bladder is now tucked into the pelvis and the peritoneum comes to lie in front. Thus, intraperitoneal forces are directed downwards on the front of the bladder (Fig. 15.9a, arrows), making prolapse unlikely.

The symphysis is approximated using a sturdy non-absorbable (0 ethibond) suture placed through the front of each pubic bone (Fig. 15.9b). An assistant grasps each thigh and approximates the pubes while the suture is tied down.

A second mattress suture is placed in front of the symphysis to reinforce the first (Fig. 15.10). The rectus muscle and its sheath are approximated in the midline with generous bites of 2/0 Vicryl.

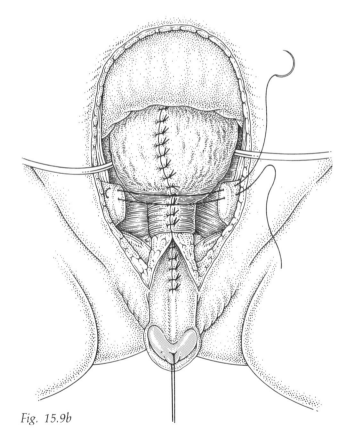

Fig. 15.9b

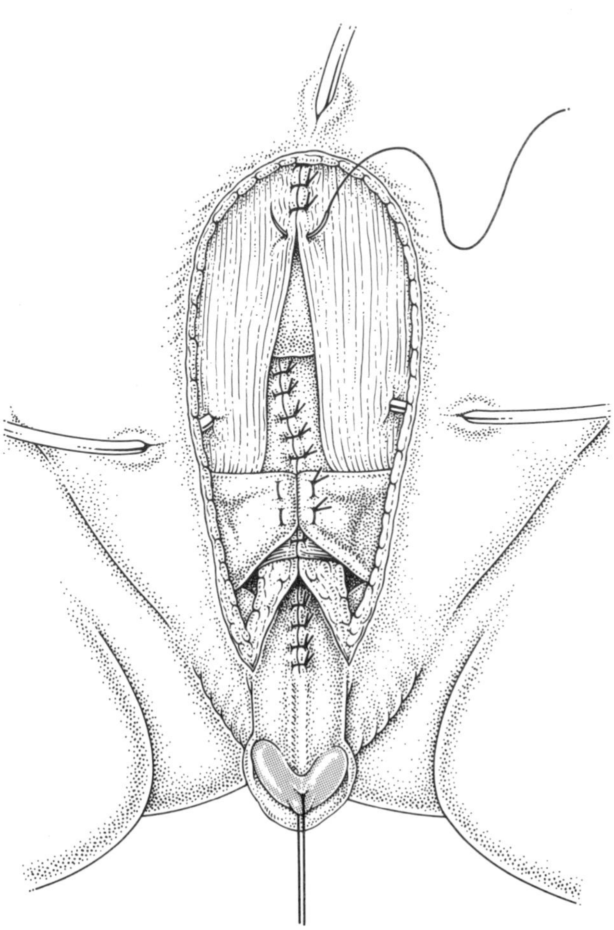

Fig. 15.10

The subcutaneous tissue and skin are closed (Fig. 15.11). Often, several more sutures are required to tubularize the neo-urethra further so as to allow it to reach the abdominal wall. No tubes or drains are left through the urethra.

The ureteric stents and a Penrose drain (not illustrated) to the perivesical space are brought out laterally. The suprapubic catheter is brought out in the midline superiorly where the umbilicus would normally be located. If a small 'x'-shaped incision is made and the apices of the flaps are turned inwards around the suprapubic catheter, a cosmetically acceptable umbilicus will result when this is removed.

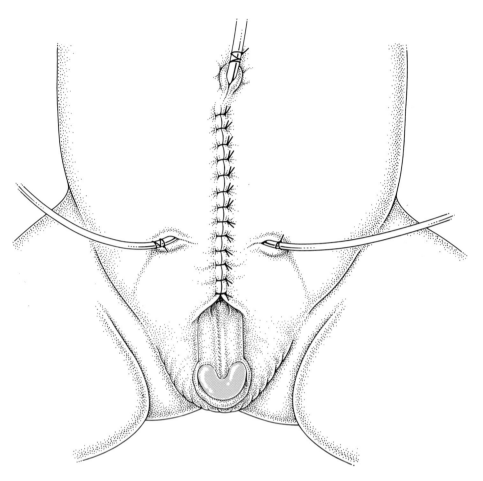

Fig. 15.11

In order to avoid stress on the closure of the symphysis, the legs are wrapped together in a 'mermaid binding'. The knees and ankles are padded with foam to prevent pressure sores and an 'Ace' wrap or crêpe bandage is used to prevent abduction of the thighs. The bandaging is re-done 2–3 times a day and maintained for 4–6 weeks.

In the older child a 'bucket handle' rectus fascial flap allows closure of the anterior abdominal wall without iliac osteo-tomies. The rectus fascia is mobilized as shown in Figure 15.12a (shaded area) and a counter incision is made trans-versely through the fascia (dotted line). As the flap is mobilized distally it is stretched between the pubic bones and is then sutured to the bone, creating a fibrous intersymphyseal band. This allows a solid reconstruction of the lower abdominal wall.

Above the rectus flap the abdominal wall is reconstructed by bringing together the rectus muscles in the midline (Fig. 15.12b). If the posterior sheath has been accidentally opened during mobilization of the rectus fascia flaps, it is important to close this during the approximation of the rectus muscles to prevent a ventral hernia. Skin closure is by lateral to medial rotational flaps.

POSTOPERATIVE CARE OF THE NEWBORN EXSTROPHY CLOSURE

Ureteric stents are maintained for 7–10 days unless drainage around them indicates that there is adequate resolution of bladder oedema to permit their safe removal. Contrast radiology up the stents prior to removal is not necessary. Two weeks postoperatively a low pressure (maximum 50 cmH$_2$O) gravity cystogram is performed to ensure that there is free bladder drainage. The suprapubic catheter may then be removed. All patients with exstrophy are presumed to have vesico-ureteric reflux and are therefore maintained on daily suppressive antibiotics. At 1 month of age an ultrasound examination of the urinary tract is performed to exclude major hydrouretero-nephrosis. At 3 months of age an intravenous urogram is performed. In the first few months after closure, a catheter is passed on a number of occasions to calibrate the neo-urethra and the bladder neck and to measure and culture residual bladder urine. An 8–10F catheter should pass easily.

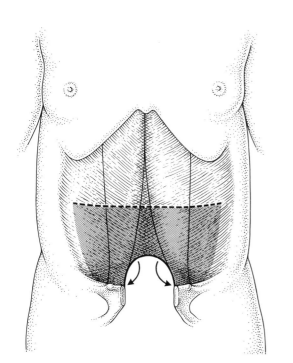

Fig. 15.12a

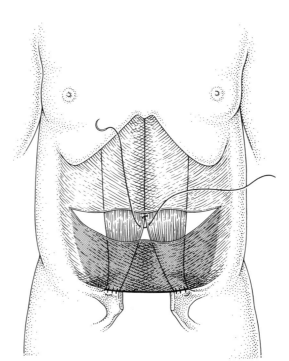

Fig. 15.12b

Male exstrophy

Second-stage genital surgery

Reconstruction of the penis following closure of a bladder exstrophy is identical to that for a mid-shaft isolated epispadias. Surgery is usually undertaken at about 12 months of age.

THE OPERATION

A urethral strip approximately 15 mm in width is isolated. On the glans the incisions are carried forward on the medial smooth superior edge so that when the glans is closed a smooth surface will result (Fig. 15.13). The incision outlining the urethral strip is continued circumferentially onto the ventrum. This will allow rotation of the ventral foreskin dorsally to provide adequate skin cover of the tubularized urethra. The glanular groove is deepened by a distal meatoplasty. A vertical incision is made from within the urethral groove almost through the glans. The vertical incision is closed transversely with interrupted 5/0 Vicryl sutures (see Fig. 15.39b, d). In this way the urethral meatus is moved ventrally to permit a glanuloplasty that does not leave the meatus on the dorsum of the glans.

The penile skin is mobilized. The skin to be tubularized as the neo-urethra is freed just sufficiently to allow closure (Fig. 15.14). Over-dissection may endanger the blood supply to the urethra. Within the glanular groove mobilization must be performed carefully as the sides of the groove are often irregular, and care must be taken to preserve sufficient healthy tissue for closure. The injection of adrenaline 1 in 100 000 helps to control bleeding.

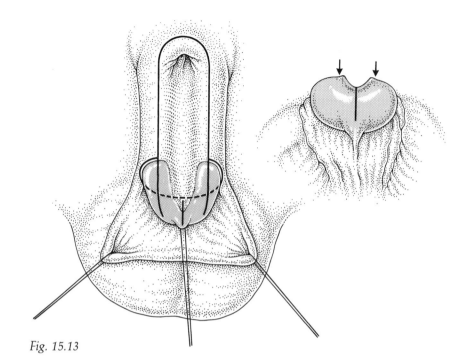

Fig. 15.13

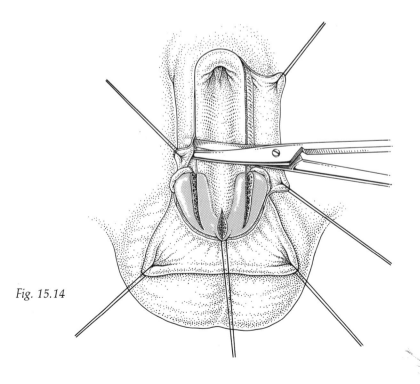

Fig. 15.14

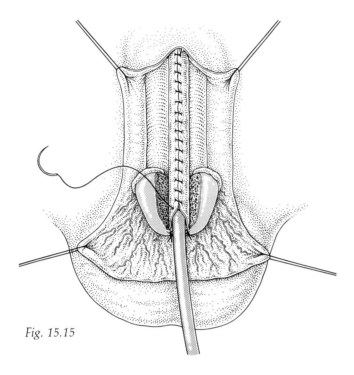

Fig. 15.15

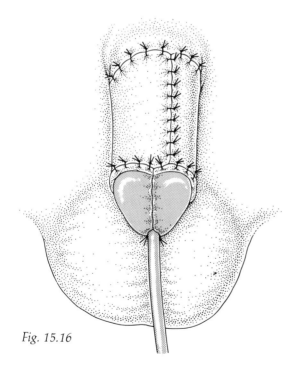

Fig. 15.16

The neo-urethra is tubularized with a continuous running inverting suture of 5/0 or 6/0 Dexon or PDS (Fig. 15.15). Glans closure is carried out in two layers. The deep layer wraps the glans comfortably around the urethra. If there is insufficient glans to be wrapped around the neo-urethra without tension, the surface of the incised glans can be opened out further by longitudinal incisions. The ventral foreskin is opened out for a reversed Byars' transfer.

The second layer of the glans closure is a subcuticular running stitch to avoid leaving suture marks on the glans (Fig. 15.16). The meatus should be at the tip of the penis with a vertical orientation and not opening dorsally in a residual epispadiac position. The reversed Byars' dorsal transfer of the ventral foreskin is completed. It is wise to build up several layers of tissue over the neo-urethra as there is a high instance of fistulas following epispadias repair, probably due to the difficulty of producing effective urinary diversion in a patient with an incompetent bladder neck. A silastic 6F urethral stent is placed through the repair and into the bladder. A monofilament suture through the stent secures it to the glans for 2 weeks.

Male exstrophy
Secondary genital surgery with division of urethral plate and reverse ventral preputial flap

The technique described in this section can be employed for primary repair of an isolated peno-pubic epispadias, but we prefer the tumble tube repair, described later, for such cases. The method has its main application as a re-operation in those boys who have undergone previous exstrophic bladder and urethral reconstruction but in whom the urethral plate has not been divided nor the prostate mobilized. The corpora cavernosa have not been adequately freed and are still tethered to the pubic bones.

THE OPERATION

This patient has already had a glans closure. The incision is made circumferentially around the meatus and dorsally down the penile shaft to the subcoronal region (Fig. 15.17). It is then carried circumferentially around the penis, keeping very close to the corporal bodies to avoid damaging the blood supply to the preputial skin. The dorsal urethral plate is usually short because the prostate has not been dropped back from its intercorporeal position.

The skin is mobilized from the corpora circumferentially (Fig. 15.18). If the prostate is still positioned distally between the corpora, it is mobilized and dropped back, permitting the corpora to become more dependent. Freeing of residual tethering of the corpora to the pubic bone may be required. If intrinsic chordee is noted on artificial erection (each corporal body must be injected separately as they do not intercommunicate), one of four options may be undertaken: (1) a Nesbit-type ventral plication of the tunica albuginea at the site of maximum curvature, (2) lateral rotation of the corporal bodies, (3) transverse incision of the tunica and medial rotation and anastomosis of the corpora (Ransley 1988), or (4) transverse incision and dermal or tunica vaginalis graft. Our preference is for the Nesbit plication to correct minor intrinsic chordee and for Ransley's repair (see later) for major chordee.

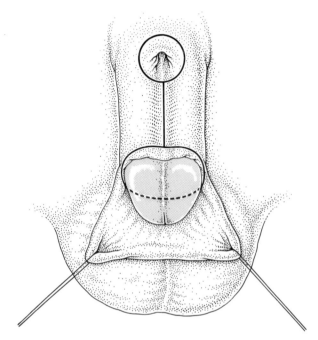

Fig. 15.17

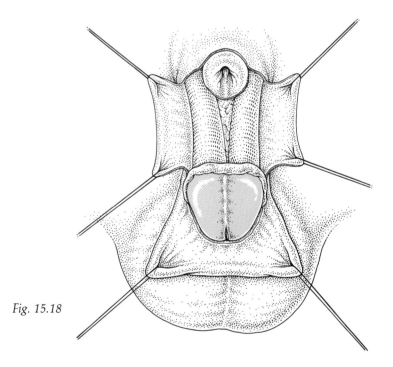

Fig. 15.18

The preparation of the ventral transverse preputial tube is a mirror image of the technique used in hypospadias repair (Chapter 17). The pedicle of the tube is mobilized from the outer ventral foreskin by dissecting parallel to the ventral foreskin, carefully sparing the intrinsic blood supply to both the island flap and the outer skin (Fig. 15.19). The preputial flap is made approximately 15 mm wide in a small boy and 20 + mm wide in a pubertal male. An inverting closure with interrupted sutures is performed.

The pedicled inner preputial tube is brought dorsally either around or between the corporal bodies (Fig. 15.20).

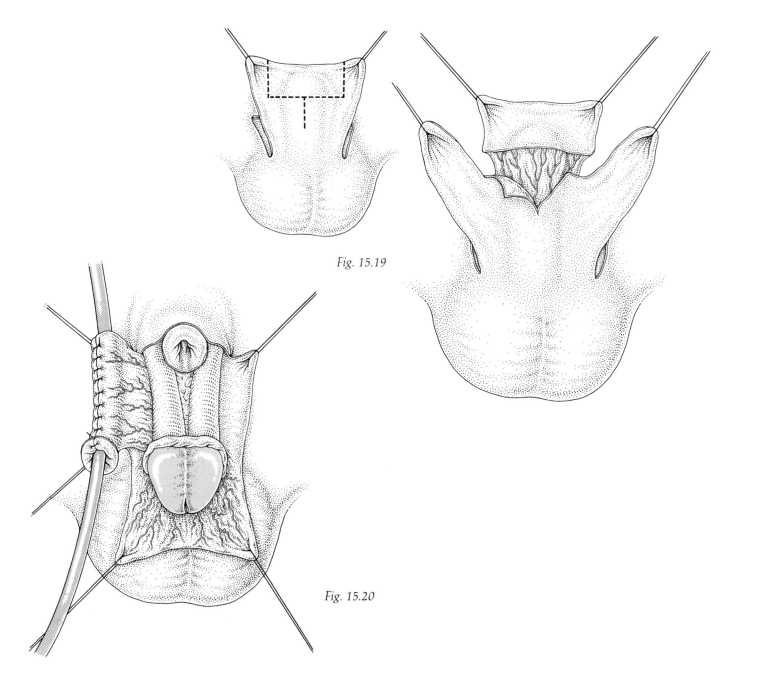

Fig. 15.19

Fig. 15.20

A spatulated anastomosis with the
suture line of the neo-urethra buried
against the corpora is performed
(Fig. 15.21). Usually the pedicle is sufficiently redundant to be tacked over the
suture lines.

Ventral residual foreskin is transferred
dorsally and closed in several layers to
complete the repair (Fig. 15.22). Urinary
diversion is by silastic stent (6F for small
boys, 8F for older children) or an 8F
silastic Foley catheter. The catheter and
stents are left in for 2 weeks.

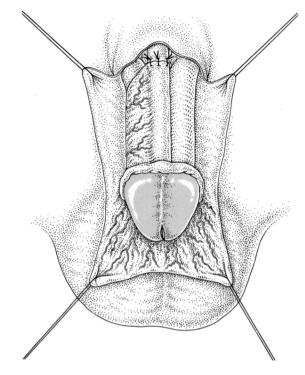

Fig. 15.21

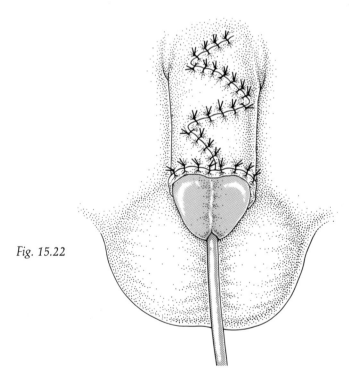

Fig. 15.22

REFERENCES

Ransley P G 1988 Epispadias repair. In: Dudley H, Carter D, Russell R C G
  (eds) Operative surgery, 4th edn. Butterworth, London, p 627–632

The Ransley second-stage urethroplasty for exstrophy

This method of repair is applicable to the older boy in whom it is anticipated that the dorsal penile chordee is due to corporal disproportion developing with growth.

THE OPERATION

The skin incisions outlining the urethral strip that will be tubularized are carried around the ventrum of the penis at the subcoronal level (Fig. 15.23a). A meatoplasty, the IPGAM (the reverse of the meatoplasty carried out in a Magpi distal hypospadias repair), is performed. A vertical incision in the urethral groove is made almost through the glans (Fig. 15.23b, c). The incision is closed transversely, widening the urethra and positioning the meatus ventrally (Fig. 15.23d).

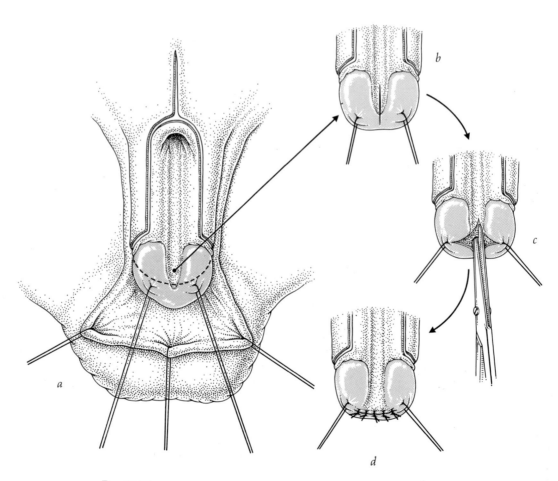

Fig. 15.23

The penile skin is mobilized completely from the corporal bodies (Fig. 15.24). Dorsal nerves, as shown in the figure, are normally only seen in the older child.

This ventral view shows the extent of the corporal mobilization (Fig. 15.25). Care must be taken not to dissect the urethral plate too widely from the subcutaneous tissues so that its blood supply is preserved. This is achieved by keeping the dissection close to the corpora, at the same time being careful not to injure the dorsal nerves.

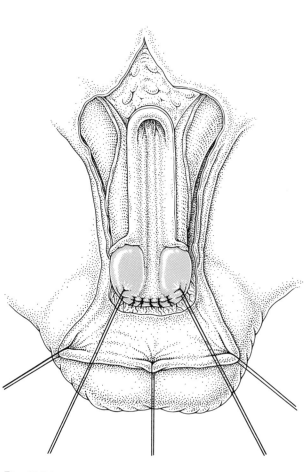

Fig. 15.24

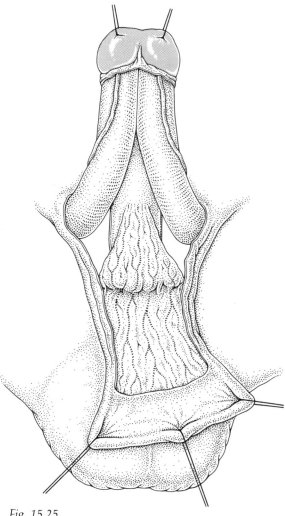

Fig. 15.25

The incisions that outlined the urethral strip are carried into the glans (Fig. 15.26). The glans wings must be adequately mobilized to permit ventral placement of the neo-urethra.

The neo-urethra is tubularized with continuous inverting Dexon or Vicryl sutures (Fig. 15.27). If the closure is watertight a fistula is less likely to develop.

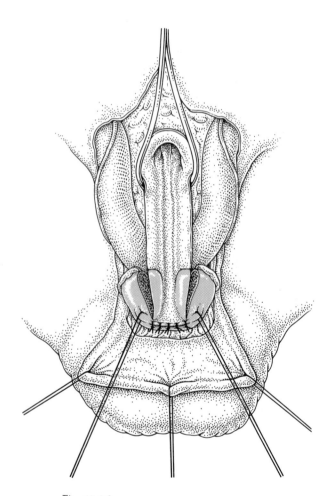

Fig. 15.26

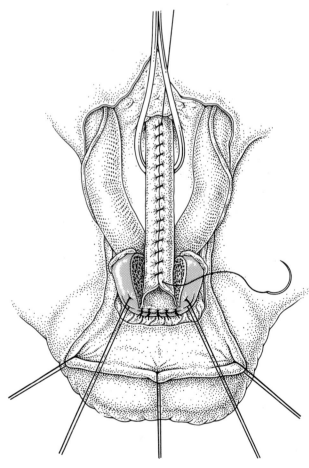

Fig. 15.27

Figure 15.28 shows the Ransley technique to correct intrinsic chordee. This procedure is most commonly required in older boys when the dorsal chordee is usually due to corporal disproportion that develops with growth. Chordee correction of this type is usually not required when the second stage urethroplasty has been carried out in the second year of life, as is our current practice at the Children's Hospital of Philadelphia.

A transverse incision is made dorsally through the tunica albuginea at the point of maximum upward bend of each corpus (Fig. 15.28a). The incision must be wide enough to completely divide the short dorsal tunica albuginea. As this is done, the transverse incisions will open out into a diamond (Fig. 15.28b), effectively lengthening the dorsal portion of the tunica albuginea and correcting the intrinsic chordee. The two diamond-shaped openings in the corpora are now anastomosed with two continuous 5/0 PDS watertight sutures (Fig. 15.28c, d). This rolls the corporal bodies medially and creates a communication between the erectile tissue of each corpus (Fig. 15.28d). Note that the urethra is positioned ventral to the anastomosis.

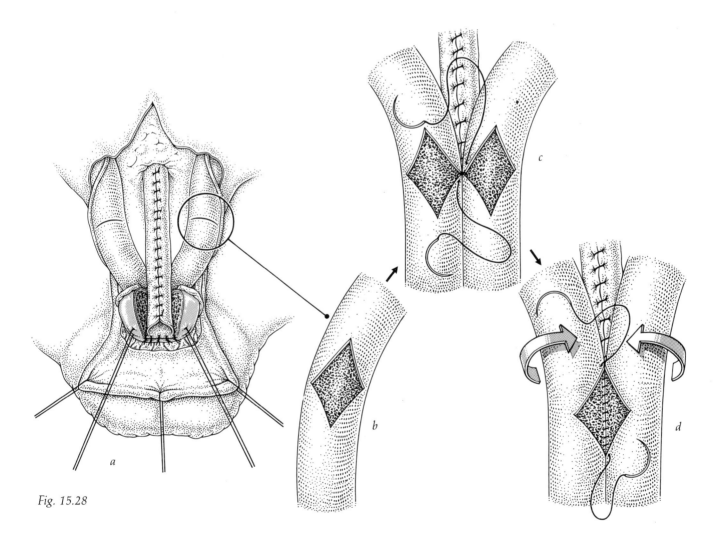

Fig. 15.28

The glanuloplasty is completed in two layers, the second layer being a subcuticular closure of the glans to minimize scarring (Fig. 15.29). Note the ventral position of the meatus, giving a correct direction of the urethra. As the corporal bodies are rotated medially, the dorsal nerves come to lie in a normal dorsal position.

An incision is made in the inner preputial layer so that an island flap of skin can be mobilized as for a hypospadias repair (Fig. 15.30). This skin flap will be rotated around the corpora to provide dorsal skin coverage.

The inner preputial flap is rotated dorsally (Fig. 15.31). The pedicle of this flap has been separated from the ventral skin in the plane immediately adjacent to the intrinsic blood supply of the ventral outer preputial skin. This preserves the pedicle as well as the vascularity of the ventral skin.

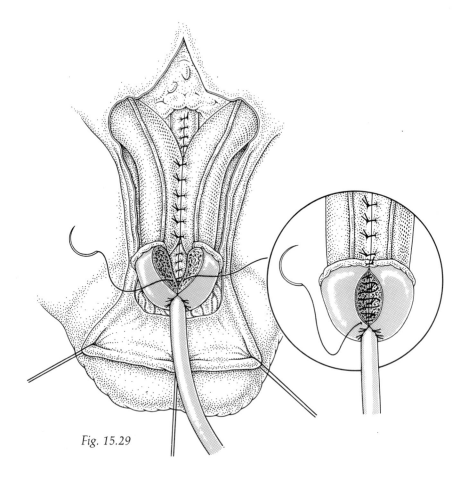

Fig. 15.29

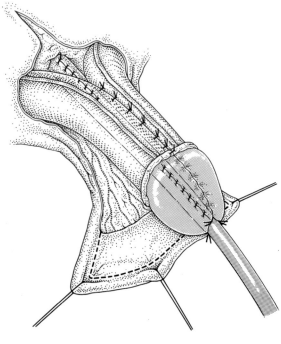

Fig. 15.30

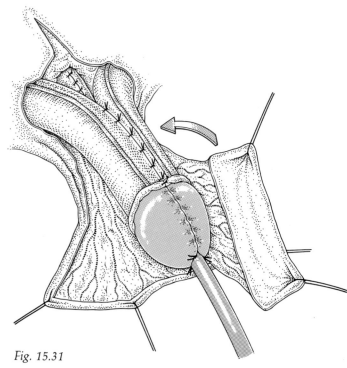

Fig. 15.31

The repair is completed. The laterally positioned skin suture lines help to prevent fistula formation (Fig. 15.32). The subcuticular glans epithelial closure gives an almost imperceptible scar. The meatus is in a ventral position on the tip of the penis, ensuring a well-directed stream.

Urinary diversion postoperatively is carried out in the same way as with the other repairs.

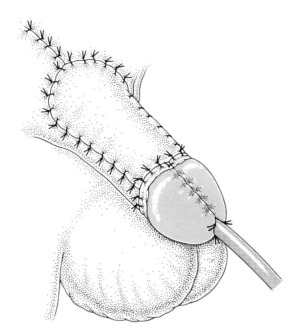

Fig. 15.32

Tumble tube repair of penopubic epispadias

THE OPERATION

Figure 15.33 shows a lateral view of isolated penopubic epispadias. The dorsal tethering of the penis is a result of the attachment of the corpora to the separated pubic bones and of the abnormal position of the prostate which lies distally between the corporal bodies and results in a shortened urethral plate.

A circumferential incision at the subcoronal level divides the urethral plate dorsally and enables the plane of dissection to be established close to the corporal bodies (Fig. 15.34). As the corpora are mobilized the prostate will be displaced proximally. The incisions for the glanuloplasty are made on the flattened top of the glans, preserving the urethral plate in the glanular groove thick enough to remain well vascularized but thin enough so that the glanular urethra can be turned in easily.

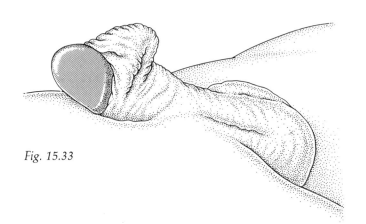

Fig. 15.33

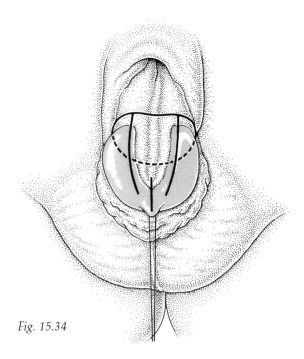

Fig. 15.34

The ventral skin of the shaft of the penis is dropped back until it is free of the corporal bodies (Fig. 15.35). Dorsally corporal mobilization is continued until the prostate is completely mobilized and the tethering of the corpora to the pubic bones is revealed (Fig. 15.36).

The urethral plate and prostate are now mobilized to expose the separated pubic bones and the fibrous bands that contribute variably to the upward angulation of the corpora. The dissection is kept against the pubic bones and continued until the corpora are no longer dorsally angulated. A periosteal elevator helps with this dissection. The deep penile vasculature in Alcock's canal must not be damaged. This is not usually a problem, as the degree of tethering once the prostate has been adequately mobilized is not usually extensive.

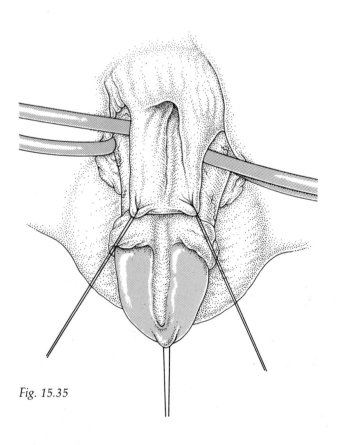

Fig. 15.35

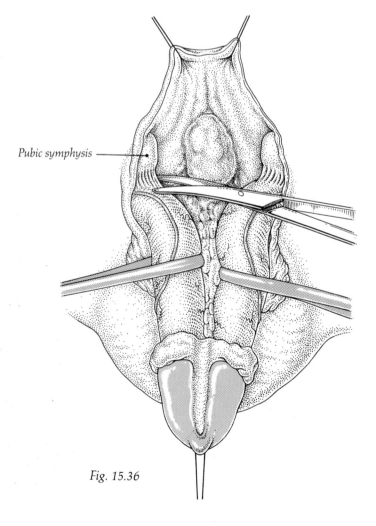

Pubic symphysis

Fig. 15.36

The ventral view in Figure 15.37 shows the mobilized skin and corporal bodies. The ventral skin can be unfolded and split as Byars' flaps for later dorsal transfer at the completion of the operation to obtain skin cover. Note the lateral position of the dorsal nerves. Although these are easily seen in the older child, in infants they are difficult to identify.

An artificial erection is induced using saline. As the two corporal bodies do not communicate, separate injections into each are required (Fig. 15.38), during which the base of the corpus is compressed against the pubic bone. Any residual bend is due to intrinsic chordee, but this is unusual when the repair is performed in early life.

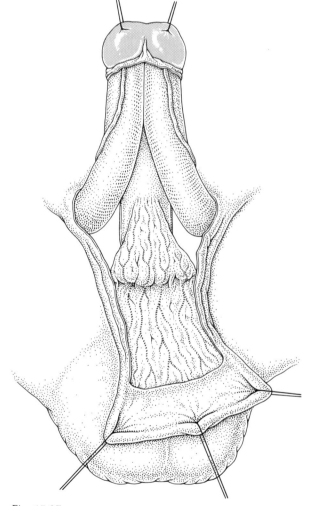

Fig. 15.37

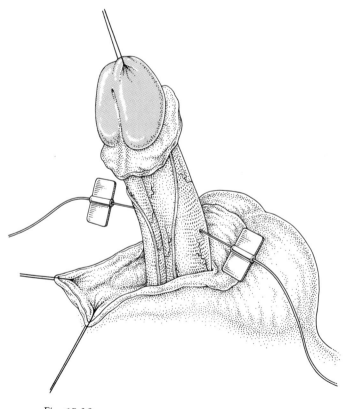

Fig. 15.38

The IPGAM procedure is used to reposition the urethral meatus ventrally. An incision is made in the glans vertically (Fig. 15.39a, b) that must be deep enough to pass almost through the complete glans. This incision is closed transversely (Fig. 15.39c, d). When the glans is closed, the meatus will be positioned ventrally to give both a normal glanular appearance and a urinary stream that can be directed normally.

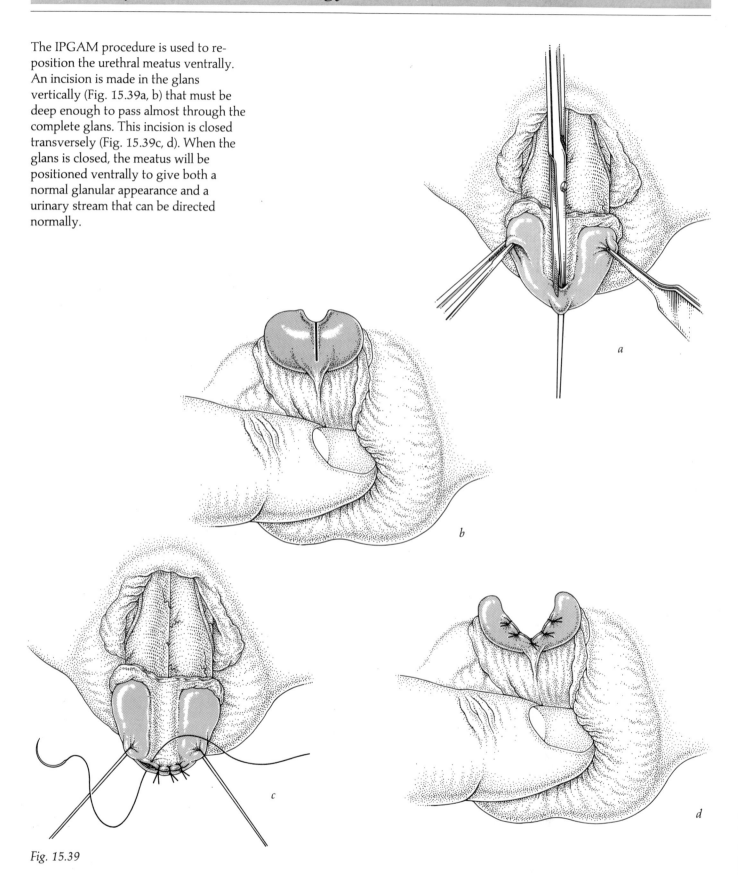

Fig. 15.39

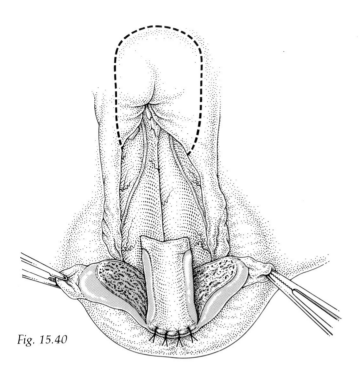

Fig. 15.40

The hairless skin above the urethral meatus is outlined (Fig. 15.40). This tumble tube flap will complete the urethroplasty. The wings of glanular tissue are adequately mobilized to allow them to be wrapped around the neo-urethra without tension. The glanular urethra is mobilized, keeping it thick enough to preserve its vascularity but thin enough to enable easy tubularization.

The tumble tube flap is mobilized (Fig. 15.41). The subcutaneous tissue must be preserved with the skin in order to help maintain a good blood supply. Tubularization of the glanular urethra with inverting sutures has been performed. The proximal end of this urethra is left spatulated so that an oblique anastomosis can be performed with the tumble tube flap.

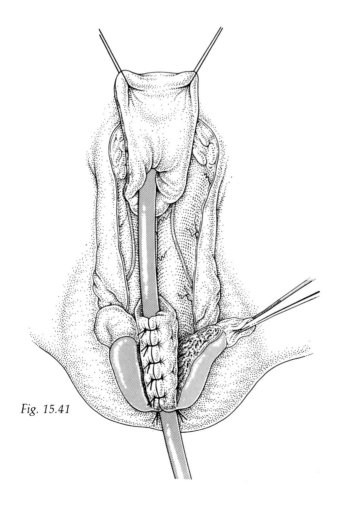

Fig. 15.41

The tumble tube flap is tubularized using inverting Dexon or Vicryl 5/0 or 6/0 sutures (Fig. 15.42). The distal end is left spatulated. Note that the suture line of the tumble tube flap will be buried against the corporal bodies.

The tumble tube flap is anastomosed to the glanular urethra using inverting interrupted sutures (Fig. 15.43). The mobilized glans wings are closed over the urethra in two layers, thus burying the urethral closure and apposing the broad surface of glans tissue.

The glans closure is completed with a subcuticular running suture (Fig. 15.44). This will result in minimal scarring on the glans. Note that the meatus is positioned ventrally to provide a well-directed urinary stream.

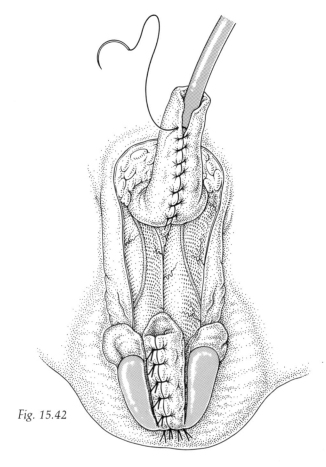

Fig. 15.42

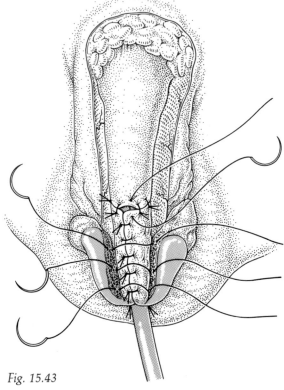

Fig. 15.43

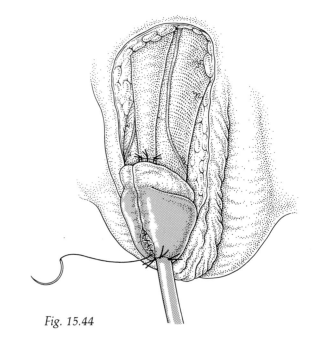

Fig. 15.44

Skin coverage is obtained by sliding around the excess ventral foreskin, using the Byar's technique (Fig. 15.45). The repair is completed with interrupted Vicryl/Dexon sutures. Note the dependent angle of the flaccid penis.

The end-on view of the healed repair in Figure 15.46 shows the correction of the dorsal tethering. The glanuloplasty has healed with a smooth surface and a thin scar. The meatus is ventrally positioned with a normal slit-like configuration.

POSTOPERATIVE CARE

An indwelling 6F silastic catheter is passed transurethrally into the bladder and sutured to the glans by a single non-absorbable monofilament suture. The urine is diverted for 2 weeks. The fistula rate is higher following an epispadias repair than a hypospadias repair, probably due to difficulty in achieving complete urinary diversion with an incompetent bladder neck.

ACKNOWLEDGEMENTS

The author wishes to acknowledge that this chapter is an assimilation of ideas and concepts garnered from many of his predecessors and colleagues in paediatric urology. Special recognition is due to Dr John Duckett, the originator of the use of paraexstrophy flaps, Sir David Innes Williams and Mr J. Herbert Johnston—the author's mentors. Mr Philip Ransley and many of the author's contemporaries have contributed to this presentation which it is hoped will be useful to future generations of paediatric urologists.

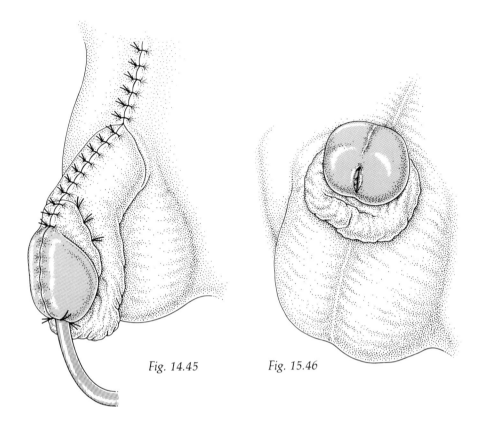

Fig. 14.45   *Fig. 15.46*

Chapter 16

Bladder neck reconstruction in the incontinent child

John P. Gearhart

Introduction

Bladder neck reconstruction in the child with incontinence remains a formidable challenge for the surgeon. Many techniques have been used in the past to achieve urinary continence. However, the timing of bladder neck surgery, the most reliable surgical procedure, the need for bladder augmentation, and optimal treatment of the child with a previously failed incontinence procedure remain controversial.

This chapter will deal with bladder neck reconstruction for the two most common causes of congenital incontinence: (1) complete epispadias and (2) classical bladder exstrophy.

BLADDER NECK RECONSTRUCTION IN COMPLETE EPISPADIAS

The attainment of satisfactory urinary continence in epispadias remains a surgical challenge. Not only is the bladder small and thin, but the trigonal-urethral canal is also severely defective. The trigone is poorly developed and the vesical neck is open, with patulous, laterally placed ureteric orifices. A vast majority of these children also have associated vesico-ureteric reflux. The rarity of this entity, when compared with the exstrophy–epispadias complex, makes a large series of these patients difficult to assemble.

BLADDER NECK RECONSTRUCTION IN EXSTROPHY

Successful bladder neck reconstruction in exstrophy patients really begins with the initial bladder closure. Ideally, this should be undertaken within 72 hours of birth but later closure, well performed, can lead to continence. In a recent review of our patients a successful initial closure of the bladder was the most important factor leading to eventual continence. Patients who developed partial dehiscence prolapse or who required re-closure did not achieve continence as often as those with initial primary healing.

TIMING OF BLADDER NECK RECONSTRUCTION

At 2 years of age, an estimate of bladder capacity is needed and may best be obtained by a cystogram and cystoscopy under anaesthesia. Other means of estimating bladder disten-sibility and capacity in the crying child may be impossible. The cystogram will measure bladder capacity and will also determine whether reflux is present. If the bladder capacity is increasing and is expected to reach 60 ml or better by the age of 3 or $3\frac{1}{2}$ years, then bladder neck reconstruction may be planned. With exstrophy, we have performed the bladder reconstruction first and then, ap-proximately 6 months later, carried out penile epispadias repair prior to bladder neck reconstruction in order to increase outlet resistance and promote bladder enlargement (Peters et al 1988, Gearhart & Jeffs 1988b). These two studies have confirmed the added capacity that one achieves by this regimen.

TYPE OF RECONSTRUCTION

Formerly, surgical procedures designed to establish continence in both males and females gave rather discouraging results. In the last few years, however, reports have shown that the Young–Dees–Leadbetter procedure (Young 1922, Dees 1949, Leadbetter 1964), or a modification thereof, offers the best probability of continence in these patients (Oesterling & Jeffs 1987).

The addition of a Marshall–Marchetti–Krantz (1949) bladder neck suspension certainly has improved the overall continence rate. Intraoperative pressure profilimetry has confirmed that the latter manoeuvre increases both the urethral closure pressure and the continence length (Gearhart et al 1986).

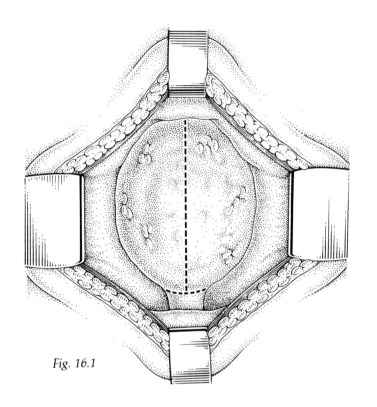

Fig. 16.1

SURGICAL TECHNIQUE

A 'U'-shaped incision is made very low on the bladder neck and the incision is extended into a midline cystotomy (Fig. 16.1). With a low 'U' incision, the bladder can retract in a cephalad manner for easy access to the bladder neck reconstruction area (Fig. 16.2).

Ureteric reimplantation is performed in a trans-trigonal manner, not only to correct reflux, but also to move the ureters away from the bladder neck so that sufficient trigonal tissue is available for bladder neck reconstruction (Fig. 16.3).

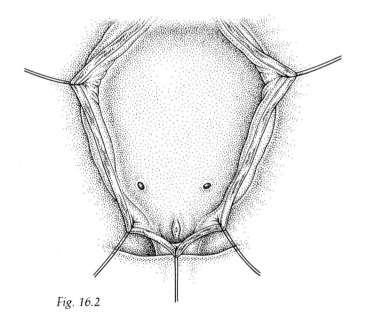

Fig. 16.2

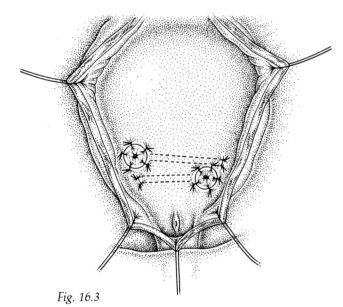

Fig. 16.3

Alternatively, the ureters can be directed more cephalad, thus allowing even greater access to the trigonal area (Fig. 16.4).

The incontinence procedure is begun by outlining a strip of mucosa approximately 18–20 mm in width by 30 mm in length that extends from the mid-trigone to the prostatic or posterior urethra (Fig. 16.5). The bladder muscle lateral to the mucosal strip is denuded of mucosa by sharp dissection.

Multiple small incisions into the bladder muscle in the area of the denuded lateral triangles allow lengthening of the bladder neck area and allow the bladder to retract into a more cephalad position (Figs 16.6, 16.7). At this juncture the actual rolling of the bladder neck into a tube is ready to begin.

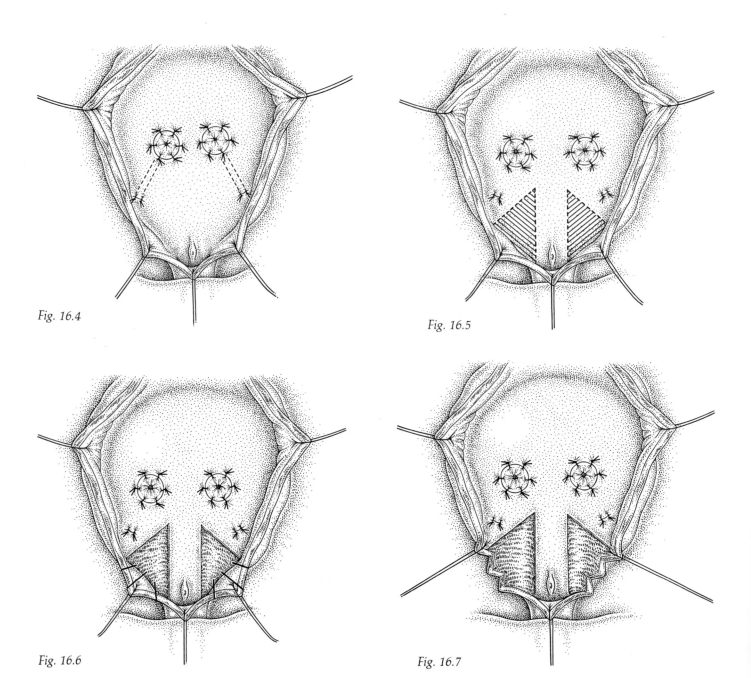

Fig. 16.4

Fig. 16.5

Fig. 16.6

Fig. 16.7

The first suture is placed at the area of the new bladder neck utilizing Vicryl or Dexon (Fig. 16.8). This stitch goes through the muscle, into the mucosa, across the midline, into the mucosa, and out again through the muscle, and is tied with a knot facing the inside of the bladder. With cephalad retraction on this stitch, the more distal areas of mucosa and the bladder neck are easily brought up into the field.

At this juncture, multiple interrupted sutures of Vicryl or Dexon, which bring some muscle along with the mucosa to the midline, are inserted (Figs 16.9, 16.10). These sutures are placed quite close together. While the innermost aspect of the bladder neck reconstruction is being performed, an 8F plastic feeding tube is left in place through the neo-urethra.

After the neo-urethral tube is constructed, the adjacent denuded muscle flaps are overlapped and sutured firmly in place in a double-breasted muscle closure of the bladder neck (Fig. 16.11). These sutures are of horizontal mattress type.

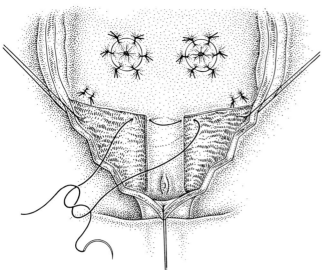

Fig. 16.8

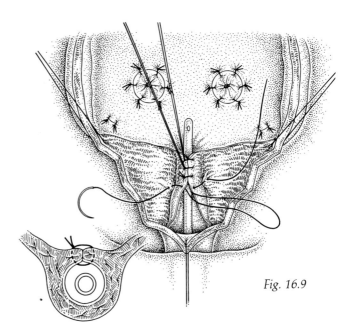

Fig. 16.9

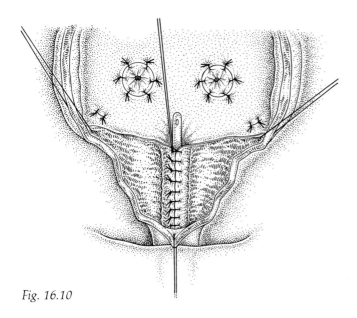

Fig. 16.10

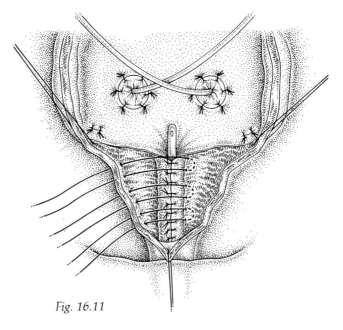

Fig. 16.11

When the second denuded muscle flap is being brought across, these sutures are intentionally left long (Fig. 16.12). The last suture at the new bladder neck and the other suture more distal to this are going to be used for suspending the bladder neck. If it is possible to leave even three of these sutures long enough for later bladder neck suspension, then all the better.

At this juncture most of the bladder reconstruction is complete except for the suspension of the newly constructed bladder neck (Fig. 16.13).

After being tubularized the bladder neck is suspended in a Marshall–Marchetti–Krantz (1949) manner through the rectus fascia to increase both the continence length and the urethral closure pressure (Fig. 16.14). Pressure profilimetry routinely reveals a closure pressure of 70–100 ml of water and a 2.5 cm continence length (Gearhart et al 1986). No indwelling stents are ordinarily left through the bladder neck reconstruction area, but if it is a re-operative reconstruction, a small 3F stent is employed. Ureteric stents are left in place for 10 days to 2 weeks and the suprapubic tube remains in place for 3 weeks.

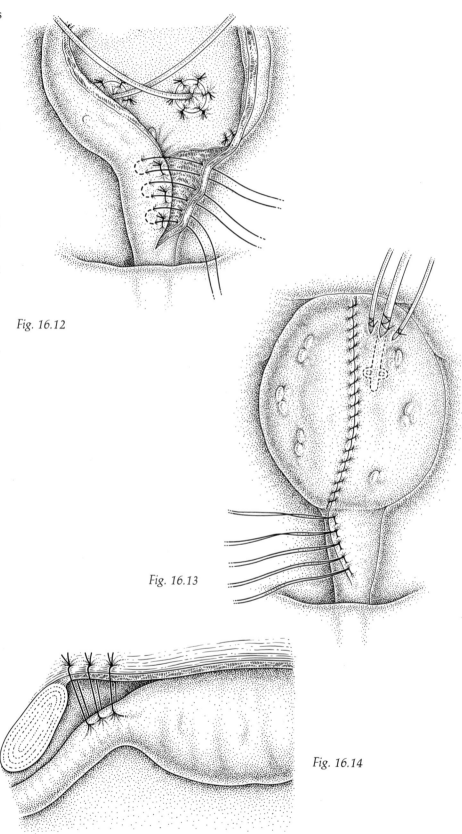

Fig. 16.12

Fig. 16.13

Fig. 16.14

POSTOPERATIVE CARE

At the end of the 3-week drainage period, the suprapubic tube is clamped and a voiding trial is attempted. If residual urines are low during the voiding trial, a 10F catheter is passed into the bladder per urethram when the child is under sedation. If there is obstruction to urine flow through the neo-urethra after 3 weeks, the suprapubic drainage may be continued and gentle urethral dilatation performed or intermittent catheterization instituted. Occasionally, a gentle cystoscopy to help 'find the way' will dilate the new urethra and the bladder neck sufficiently to allow voiding without damaging the newly constructed continence mechanism. Often, a gentle cystoscopy followed by a short period of urethral catheter (8 or 10F) drainage will dilate the neo-urethra just enough to allow voiding.

After the ureteric stents are removed but prior to removal of the suprapubic tube, an intravenous pyelogram is obtained to document adequate drainage of the upper urinary tract. The initial bladder capacity is usually quite small due to the operative procedure. However, if the child has an initial dry interval of 10–15 minutes, then the long-term chances of success are quite good. Severe urinary frequency is often a problem after bladder neck reconstruction. Urine cultures are obtained prior to suprapubic tube removal to ensure sterility of the urine, and suppressive chemotherapy is continued for 4 months postoperatively. If the cultures are negative and the urinary frequency is bothersome, imipramine in doses of 10 mg two or three times daily will often control the symptom. Usually after 4–6 weeks this dosage can be lessened, and later the drug is discontinued.

An intravenous pyelogram is obtained 4–6 months postoperatively. The urine must be kept sterile and residual urines must be monitored, initially by ultrasound and later by follow-up intravenous pyelogram. A cystogram in a well child is deferred for a year or more.

Gradually, over a period of 3–18 months, the dry interval lengthens, voiding volume increases, awareness of filling improves and detrusor function may be voluntarily controlled. Nocturia and enuresis frequently persist after daytime control is achieved, but will improve with increased capacity and maturity in sleep patterns. Suppressive chemotherapy is continued for 6–12 months or beyond if necessary while satisfactory drainage, storage and bladder function are being established.

Parent and patient education is continually required as well as personal supervision and encouragement by the surgeon. The timing of achievement of bladder and bowel control in the normal child is variable and is subject to many psychological, physiological and environmental influences. The child born with congenital incontinence must contend with anatomical deficiency, the surgical repair, physiological differences and markedly exaggerated psychological and environmental influences. However, with cooperation and time, urinary continence is an achievable goal in the majority of patients born with congenital urinary incontinence.

FAILED BLADDER NECK RECONSTRUCTION

Although the Young–Dees–Leadbetter type repair is a very reliable procedure when well performed, occasionally children are seen where an attempt has been made and has failed. Urinary diversion at this juncture is not recommended. The author believes that all such patients can be made dry if the surgeon persists and is not discouraged easily. In order to make the child dry one must have a bladder of adequate volume, the pressure in the bladder must not be too high, and there must be enough resistance in the urethra and bladder neck to exceed the pressure in the bladder during normal activity. In order to void, the child must be able to generate enough pressure in the bladder by detrusor activity or by straining to exceed the outlet resistance. Lacking this, the child must be able to empty the bladder by intermittent catheterization. These goals can usually be met in most patients with reconstructive techniques that are available today.

When presented with a child who has a failed former bladder neck reconstruction, a complete work-up is in order, including urodynamic studies, cystography, cystoscopy and upper tract evaluation. If there is low outlet resistance, then this must be increased. If the bladder volume and compliance are decreased, then the bladder capacity must be augmented. Whenever a patient presents with this type of incontinence problem, we make it very clear to the family that it may be necessary to catheterize intermittently, temporarily or even, in some cases, permanently. This is especially true if there is a small capacity bladder which must be augmented at the time of re-operative bladder neck reconstruction. Often, if the bladder capacity is adequate, a repeat Young–Dees–Leadbetter operation is the procedure of choice.

With a small capacity bladder, bladder augmentation along with reimplantation of the ureters either into the bladder patch or the selected bowel segment may be in order. As with other reconstructive procedures the bowel segment chosen should be detubularized prior to augmenting the bladder (Gearhart & Jeffs 1988a). Our results utilizing the artificial urinary sphincter in patients who have failed initial bladder neck reconstruction have not been rewarding.

REFERENCES

Dees J E 1949 Congenital epispadias with incontinence. Journal of Urology
62: 513
Gearhart J P, Jeffs R D 1988a Augmentation cystoplasty in the failed
exstrophy reconstruction. Journal of Urology 139: 790
Gearhart J P, Jeffs R D 1988b Exstrophy; the small bladder after initial
closure. American Academy of Pediatrics (abstract 21)
Gearhart J P, Williams K A, Jeffs R D 1986 Intraoperative urethral pressure
profilimetry as an adjunct to bladder neck reconstruction. Journal of
Urology 136: 1055
Leadbetter G W 1964 Surgical correction of total urinary incontinence.
Journal of Urology 91: 261
Marshall V F, Marchetti A A, Krantz K E 1949 Congenital abnormalities of
the bladder. In: Handbuch der Urologie. Springer-Verlag, New York,
p 165–218
Oesterling J E, Jeffs R D 1987 The importance of a successful initial bladder
closure in the surgical management of classical bladder exstrophy:
analysis of 144 patients treated at the Johns Hopkins Hospital between
1975 and 1985. Journal of Urology 137: 258
Peters C A, Gearhart J P, Jeffs R D 1988 Epispadias and incontinence: the
challenge of the small bladder. Journal of Urology 140: 1199–1201
Young H H 1922 An operation for the cure of incontinence associated with
epispadias. Journal of Urology 7: 1

Chapter 17

Hypospadias repair

John W. Duckett

Introduction

Since hypospadias occurs in 1 in 300 male births, its repair is a very common paediatric urological procedure. In general, upper urinary tract anomalies are not common and investigation is not required. The more severe the placement of the meatus, the more likely a large prostatic utricle will be present. This entity generally does not cause a problem except for placement of a catheter through the urethra. Nine per cent of hypospadias patients have undescended testes, and 9% have inguinal hernias or hydroceles. Of course the presence of other associated anomalies, such as a cardiac defect, imperforate anus, tracheo-oesophageal fistula, etc., would require a more extensive urological investigation.

After 20 years' experience of repairing hypospadias, the present author is confining his diagrams and remarks to those techniques used at the Children's Hospital of Philadelphia. The classification used is the location of the meatus after the release of chordee. Thus, anterior hypospadias contributes about 65% of cases, middle hypospadias 15% of cases, and posterior hypospadias 20% of cases.

Techniques used for anterior hypospadias are: (1) MAGPI, (2) extended MAGPI, (3) Mathieu and (4) onlay transverse preputial island flap. Techniques used for middle hypospadias are: (1) onlay island flap and (2) transverse preputial island flap urethroplasty. Techniques used for posterior hypospadias are: (1) transverse preputial island flap urethroplasty, (2) transverse preputial island flap plus perineal extension and (3) double-faced island flap. The final group is complex re-do hypospadias repair. A variety of techniques are utilized including bladder mucosal free-graft urethroplasty.

MEATAL ADVANCEMENT AND GLANULOPLASTY (MAGPI)
(Fig. 17.1)

The most common lesion is a sub-coronal meatus with a blind-ending distal groove. The stream is deflected ventrally by 45 degrees. In about one-third of cases, the meatus is very stenotic. A dorsal preputial hood is present with a median raphe deviating off to one side, causing penile torsion to the left. Frequently, the skin on the ventrum is very thin and tethering. There is apparent chordee in many of these cases but, after skin release, an artificial erection will reveal a straight penis. It is inappropriate to judge the presence of chordee prior to release of skin tethering.

To flatten out the skin bridge distal to the meatus, a vertical incision is made into the glanular groove for about 1 cm (Fig. 17.1b, c, d). This creates a diamond-shaped defect which is closed transversely with 6/0 or 7/0 chromic catgut. This effectively opens the meatus, flattens the groove, and advances the dorsal meatal edge into the glans.

The glanuloplasty portion is formed by elevating the ventral meatal edge forward (Fig. 17.1f). Two holding stitches are placed on the glanular wings which are brought ventrally. Redundant skin in the midline is excised so that glanular tissue can be approximated in the normal conical anatomy. Vicryl and chromic catgut are used for closure of the glans (Fig. 17.1g, h).

Generally, a sleeve re-approximation for skin cover is accomplished, but if there is significant skin deficiency, Byars' flaps must be utilized as depicted in Figure 17.2c, d.

A vaseline gauze dressing is applied which is removed the following day. No stent is required, nor a catheter for diversion. The preferred age for operation is 6 months to 1 year.

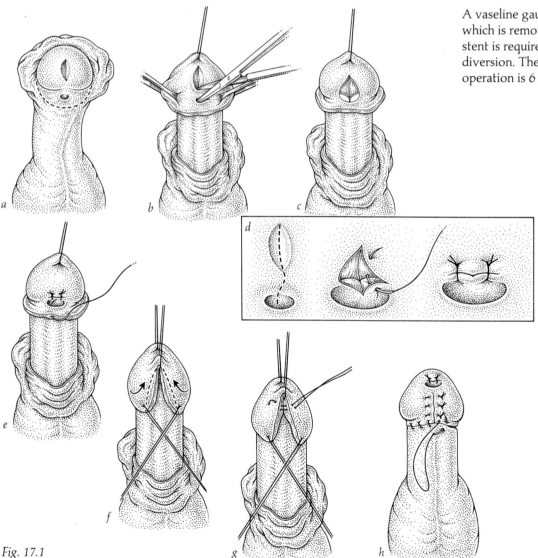

Fig. 17.1

MATHIEU PROCEDURE (PARAMEATAL-BASED FLAP)
(Figure 17.2)

This technique is utilized for the distal meatus that is about 1 cm from the corona, but is wide open and fixed so that it cannot be mobilized onto the glans with a MAGPI technique. These cases must not have any chordee. The ventral skin must be thick so that the parameatal-based flap will have adequate blood supply for mobilization and extension. The subcutaneous tissue should be left attached to the ventral flap to assure this.

The dotted lines (Fig. 17.2a) outline the skin flaps. The glans wings are approximated together to create a conical glans configuration (Fig. 17.2c). Skin coverage for this technique is often very difficult. Depicted in the diagram is the Byars' ventral rotation (Fig. 17.2c, d) which is most often utilized. It is because of the skin coverage that we generally prefer an onlay island flap technique for such a meatal configuration.

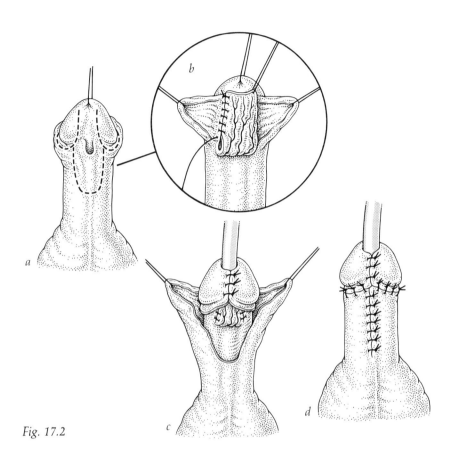

Fig. 17.2

TRANSVERSE PREPUTIAL ISLAND FLAP URETHROPLASTY WITH GLANS CHANNEL (Fig. 17.3)

This technique is universally useful for one-stage procedures in which chordee release is done at the same time as urethroplasty. It is reserved for urethral replacement of approximately 2.5—5 cm in length by having a vascularized neo-urethra. Healing proceeds without the need for revascularization from the skin cover, as is required in free skin grafts. The circumferential incision around the corona (Fig. 17.3a, b) should be made as proximal as possible to leave a good glans cap of tissue. The urethra and shaft skin are dissected free of the corpora cavernosa to release chordee tethering. It is sometimes necessary to take dorsal tucks on either side of the neurovascular bundle in order to completely correct a ventral bend to the shaft.

Once the shaft is free of chordee, demonstrated by artificial erection, the proximal native urethra is brought to a comfortable position on the shaft and fixed with 7/0 Vicryl to the tunica albuginea. The skin of the urethral meatus should be excised back to good spongiosal tissue (Fig. 17.3c).

Mobilization of the transverse preputial island flap (as depicted in Fig. 17.3d, e, f) is done in such a way as to develop a midline pedicle which is mobilized all the way down to the base of the penis. This can be done with lateral dissections also so that the base of the pedicle is narrowed and will not rotate the penis as it is spiralled around to the ventrum. The plane for this dissection is very delineated, leaving most of the vasculature to the flap itself. Since the distal extent of the penile skin will be excised, it is not a problem to have adequately vascularized penile skin for coverage.

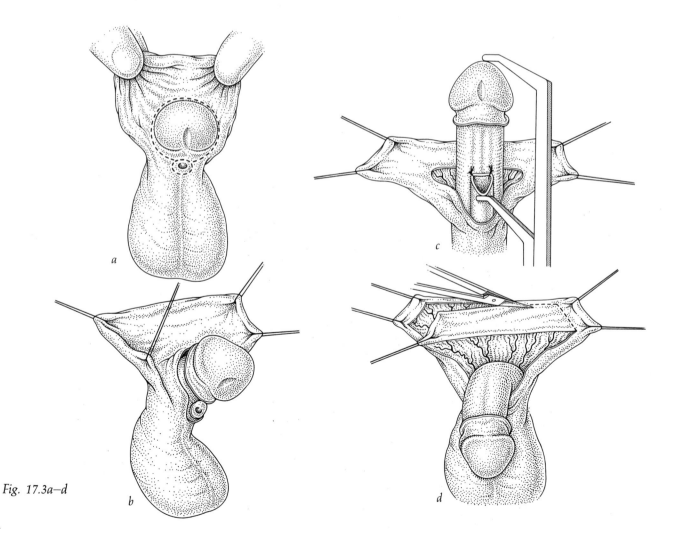

Fig. 17.3a—d

The inner transverse preputial island flap is tubularized and fashioned in such a way as to create a 12F calibre neo-urethra (Fig. 17.3f). The edges are rolled inwards with Lembert-type sutures. The ends of the tube are by interrupted sutures and the middle portion may be by a running suture if desired. This permits trimming off of the ends to tailor the urethroplasty.

The pedicle and the tube are spiralled around to the ventrum (Fig. 17.3g, h). The proximal anastomosis is done in an open fashion so that careful approximation of the edges against the fixed proximal urethra may be accomplished (Fig. 17.3g). The anastomosis is covered by the pedicle. The opposite edge of the pedicle may be tethered and may thus cause torsion. This should be relieved by careful dissection, avoiding disturbing the vasculature to the pedicle.

A glans channel is made by dissecting flat against the tunica albuginea of the corpora out to the tip of the glanular groove so that a generous channel sized 16—18F is created. Glanular tissue itself must be removed to make this channel adequate in size. It is not enough to stretch the channel since it will contract back down and compress the blood supply of the pedicle as it lies in the glans channel (Fig. 17.3h). This is the most common cause of technical error in the procedure and can lead to the disastrous consequence of a strictured glanular urethra.

Once the neo-urethra is in the appropriate position, skin cover is obtained by splitting the dorsal preputial skin and bringing around flaps to the ventrum as depicted in Figure 17.3i.

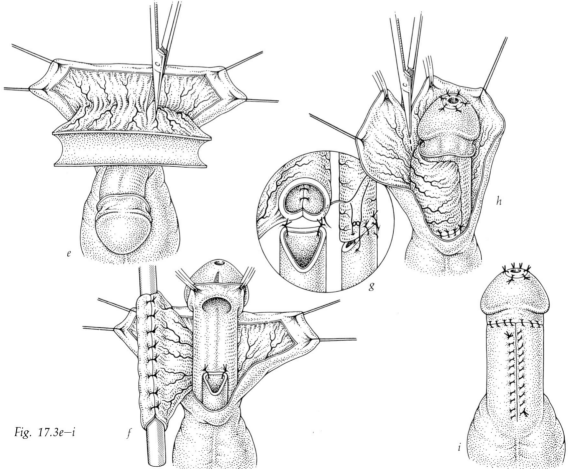

Fig. 17.3e–i

Figure 17.4 depicts another variation of transposing the transverse preputial island flap to the ventrum by button-holing the pedicle. This is done with a very long neo-urethra in severe cases where compromising the pedicle would be a problem.

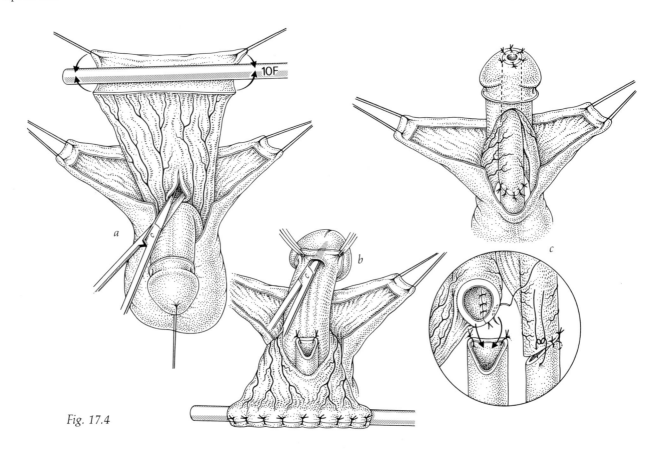

Fig. 17.4

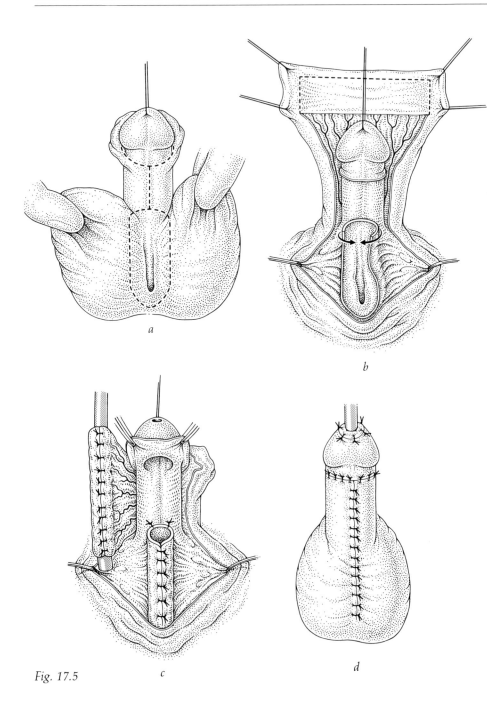

Figure 17.5 depicts a perineal extension of the urethra which may be made for very proximal perineal openings. The surrounding shiny skin can be tubularized in a Duplay fashion (Fig. 17.5a, b, c), extending the proximal urethra up to the penoscrotal area. The island flap is then rotated in the standard fashion and anastomosed to this proximal extension. Since one would like to avoid this proximal extension, it is frequently possible to anastomose the meatal portion of the tube first and stretch this down to the perineum in such a way that most of the proximal extension can be discarded.

a

b

c

d

Fig. 17.5

DOUBLE-FACED ISLAND FLAP
(Fig. 17.6)

This modification of the standard island flap technique permits dorsal preputial skin to remain attached to the pedicle in a double-faced fashion. When this is spiralled around to the ventrum, the skin still attached to the neo-urethra can be used for skin cover. It makes up one-third of the cylinder of the shaft, while the dorsal penile skin will cover the remaining two-thirds. This is particularly advantageous in epispadias repair where a reverse preputial island flap is made so that skin cover on the shaft of the epispadiac penis is enhanced with this method.

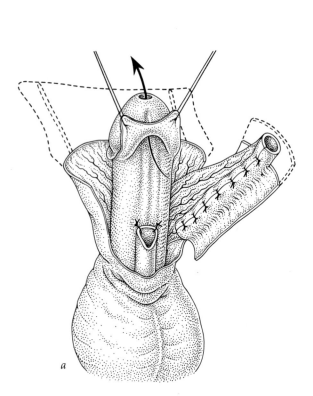

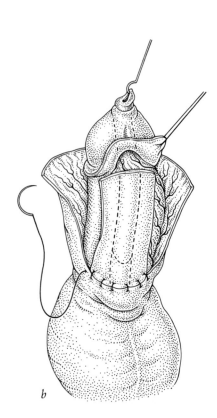

Fig. 17.6

ONLAY ISLAND FLAP (Fig. 17.7)

This procedure is for cases where the proximal meatus has a distal urethral plate of good quality. It is utilized only when there is no chordee after release of all the skin. A strip of urethral plate is outlined about 6–8 mm in width out to the tip of the penis extended on either side of the glanular groove (Fig. 17.7a). The proximal urethra is cut back to good spongiosol tissue (Fig. 17.7c). An onlay of a preputial island flap is then accomplished, making a parallel running suture line from the edge of the meatus out to the tip of the glans, rotating the half of an island flap over to the other side with a parallel suture line running up the other side (Fig. 17.7c, d, e).

Around the proximal meatus, interrupted sutures are used and fashioned in such a way that the proximal opening is calibrated at 12–14F. In this modification, it is important to trim the onlay flap to make sure that redundancy does not exist. This is assisted with calibration using bougies-à-boule. By extending the meatus out to the tip of the glans in a similar way to a Mathieu technique, glanular wings can be brought around, forming a normal conical configuration (Fig. 17.7e). Skin cover is achieved in the usual fashion.

This technique has been utilized more and more in recent years for the proximal meatus where the urethral plate is well formed. It is surprising how many times, after careful dissection of the penile skin, the penis will be perfectly straight on artificial erection, leaving the urethral plate intact. If only a small bend exists, dorsal tucks will alleviate this.

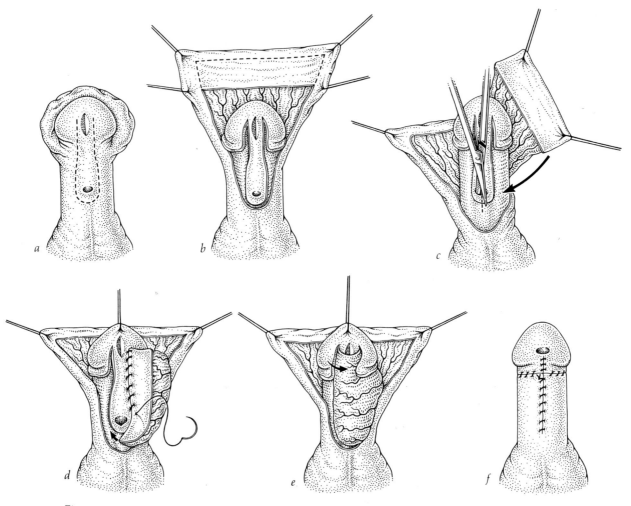

Fig. 17.7

POINTS OF TECHNIQUE AND MANAGEMENT

Magnification

We find optical loupes or Optivisor quite satisfactory. The optical microscope provides too much magnification to be helpful.

Age

We now prefer to operate on our children at 6–18 months of age, most commonly between 6 and 12 months.

Sutures

Polyglycolic or PDS 6/0 to 7/0 are normally used on the internal structures such as the neo-urethra, whereas 7/0 chromic catgut is our preferred suture for the skin and meatus.

Instruments

Ophthalmic instruments such as Castroviejo needle holders and forceps (0.5 mm), iris scissors and fine plastic needle holders are essential.

Diversion

We use a 6F silastic stent which goes all the way through the repair and into the bladder for 1 cm. A 5/0 prolene stitch is used to suture the stent to the meatus and glans. About 3–4 cm are left protruding from the tip of the penis, and urine drips continuously into the diaper. Occasionally a stent will become plugged, but the patient will void around it without difficulty. Home care of the stent is very easy. For the older child we prefer this drainage so much that we will put him into diapers for the 2 weeks that the stent is in place. This is tolerated satisfactorily as long as the child understands ahead of time.

Dressing

In the past, we used silastic foam dressings* but these are no longer available. Therefore, a Telfa pad over the repair with a bio-occlusive dressing such as Op-Site or Tegederm will suffice. The dressing is left for only 3–4 days and is removed in the office or at home. No further dressing is left after that.

Outpatient surgery

All of our patients are now operated on as day cases. The parents are very happy to take the children home, but if they come from some distance we will keep them in a nearby hotel for a day or two of observation. The patient and parents are well trained ahead of time as to what to expect in home care. Tylenol* or Tylenol plus codeine usually suffices for discomfort.

We give B & O* suppositories which are divided into thirds for bladder spasms as necessary at home.

In addition, we give Septra, one teaspoon a day, for suppression of infection in the open drainage tube. This is continued twice a day for 3 days after removal of the tube to cover any residual infection. We have not had problems with urinary tract infections with this policy of open drainage.

* Silastic foam dressings are still available in the UK (Dow Corning Corporation). Tylenol is similar to a paracetemol elixir. B & O suppositories are a mixture of belladona and opium and are not available in the UK.

Postoperative follow-up

We see the patients 4–6 days after surgery to remove the dressing and again in 10–14 days to remove the stent. Two weeks after that, the patient returns for an evaluation of the meatus and proximal anastomosis with a bougie-à-boule probing. This is not considered a dilatation, but is a calibration to make sure that there are no narrow spots. If the proximal anastomosis cannot be traversed at this visit, no dilatation or stretching is carried out unless the patient is truly obstructed. The patient returns 6 weeks later for an additional calibration and is seen again at 1-year, 3-year and 6-year intervals.

Chapter 18

Urethral reconstruction—the use of free grafts

Terry W. Hensle
Kevin A. Burbige

Introduction

Our ability to do major urethral reconstructions has been greatly enhanced by the use of both free and vascularized full-thickness grafts of local genital skin. As a general rule, whenever local genital skin is available, it should be preferentially used for urethral reconstruction and penile repair. Unfortunately, at times we are faced with patients in whom insufficient acceptable genital skin is available. Typically this is a patient in whom there have been several previous operative procedures and who is left not only with little usable local skin but also with extensive scarring. Attempts to utilize local flap and pedicle techniques in this type of patient with ischaemic tissues are likely to produce poor results. In instances such as these, where local tissue is inadequate for urethral repair, one is forced to turn to grafts from distant sites. Free grafts of full- and split-thickness skin as well as bladder mucosa are presently most frequently utilized in these difficult salvage situations.

RECIPIENT SITE

Regardless of the technique chosen for urethral reconstruction, proper preliminary preparation of the recipient site cannot be emphasized too strongly. Residual chordee is frequently encountered and is most often due to scarring from previous operative procedures. Thorough excision of all ischaemic skin and scar tissue is needed to ensure a straight penis and a healthy, well-vascularized recipient site. Remaining neo-urethra from previous repairs should also be sacrificed if there is any question as to its viability. During the initial stages of healing, a graft is nourished by passive inbibing of plasma and tissue fluids, and in the later stages an actual penetration of new capillaries into the graft occurs (Converse & Brauer 1964). Split-thickness skin grafts do not require such a well-vascularized recipient site as do full-thickness grafts due to the greater number of vessel openings on the graft undersurface. This may be of importance in a re-operative situation when one is dealing with a compromised recipient field.

SKIN GRAFTS

Both split-thickness and full-thickness free skin grafts have been utilized for urethral reconstruction, and each has its advantages and disadvantages. When considering the donor site one should choose an area of relatively hairless skin to avoid the so-called 'urethral beard' which can promote calculi formation. While individuals may vary in their degree of hirsutism, the most reliable hairless donor sites are the inner aspect of the upper arm, the post-auricular area, the eyelid and the buttock. If the urethral defect is large, two small grafts from these sites may be joined together.

Split-thickness skin grafts

Nove-Josserand (1897) first reported his results using split-thickness skin grafts for urethral reconstruction. His follow-up report (Nove-Josserand 1914) noted a high incidence of graft contracture, and the procedure fell into disuse until revived by McIndoe (1937). Since that time, improved surgical technique and a better understanding of how graft healing occurs have increased its reliability so that the technique remains useful today.

Split-thickness skin grafts are termed thin (0.005–0.012 in), medium (0.012–0.018 in) and thick (0.018–0.028 in) depending on the amount of deep dermis included with the graft. While there are many factors involved in the healing of both full- and split-thickness skin grafts, experimental studies and clinical experience have indicated that the deep dermal elements included in the graft are probably the most important determinants in pre-venting graft contraction (Corps 1969). Since human skin varies in thickness throughout the body, it is not the absolute thickness of the graft that is im-portant but its relative thickness as compared with the donor site that determines the amount of dermis included. The skin thickness of the inner upper arm in the adult male is approximately 0.046 inches, so that 0.020 inch split-thickness skin graft will include sufficient dermal elements to prevent significant contraction such as was reported in the older literature, where only thin grafts were utilized (Young & Benjamin 1949).

Full-thickness skin grafts

Humby (1941) described a one-stage hypospadias repair using a full-thickness skin graft. McCormack (1954) revived interest in full-thickness skin grafts for urethral reconstruction and the technique has been popularized by Devine & Horton (1961). The theoretical advantage of a full-thickness graft is that it includes all deep dermal elements needed to ensure proper healing and prevent graft contracture.

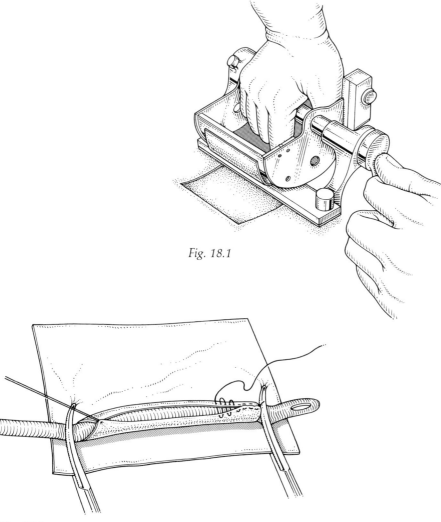

Fig. 18.1

Fig. 18.2

Surgical technique

The urethral defect to be bridged or replaced is measured with calipers and an area approximately 1.5 times the length of the measured defect is outlined on the donor site with a skin marker. The extra length is used to allow for shrinkage of the graft with handling. The width of the graft is chosen to comply with appropriate urethral diameter for the age of the patient.

If a split-thickness graft is utilized, we prefer to harvest it with the Reese dermatome because of the accuracy with which the graft thickness can be obtained (Fig. 18.1). The outlined area on the donor site is painted with liquid adhesive and allowed to dry. When the dermatome drum is placed against this area, the skin will adhere to it, allowing the knife to cut only adherent skin. If a full-thickness skin graft is chosen, the graft is excised along the outlined area with a scalpel and its undersurface carefully defatted.

The graft is then tubularized (epithelial surface inwards) over an appropriately sized fenestrated catheter with a running 6/0 absorbable suture (Fig. 18.2). Care is taken to invert the skin edges to minimize the risk of fistula formation.

The proximal urethral opening is circumscribed and freed from the surrounding skin (Fig. 18.3).

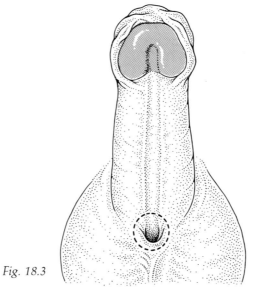

Fig. 18.3

A tunnel is created by blunt forceps dissection from the proximal meatus distally through which the neo-urethra will be placed (Fig. 18.4).

After freshening its edges, the proximal urethra is spatulated dorsally to provide a widely patent anastomosis. The graft is drawn into place (Fig. 18.5), ensuring that the suture line lies dorsally against the corpora cavernosa, and the anastomosis is then performed using individual 6/0 absorbable sutures.

The external urethral meatus is fashioned at the tip of the penis. An indwelling fenestrated catheter traversing the anastomosis is positioned (Fig. 18.6).

Urinary diversion is provided either by a perineal urethrostomy or by a suprapubic cystostomy, and an occlusive dressing is left undisturbed for 10 days.

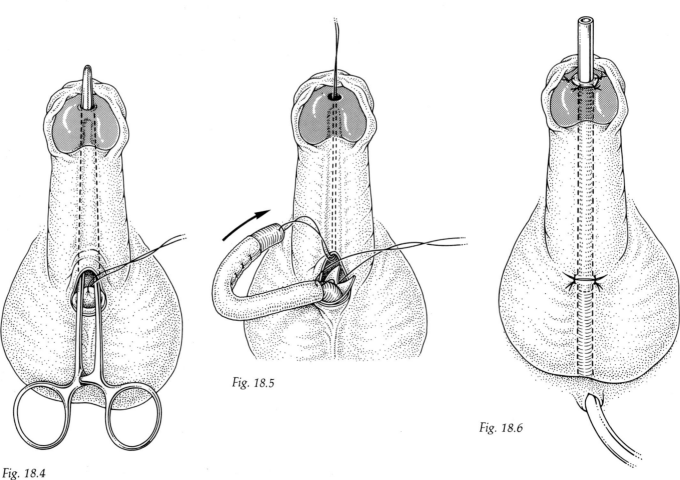

Fig. 18.4

Fig. 18.5

Fig. 18.6

BLADDER MUCOSAL GRAFTS

Memmelaar (1947) first described a one-stage repair of penoscrotal hypospadias utilizing bladder mucosa. Marshall & Spellman (Marshall 1955, Marshall & Spellman 1957) reported their results with a two-stage technique, also utilizing bladder mucosa, for construction of a neo-urethra; however, the rates of anastomotic stricture and fistula were high and the method was largely abandoned. With improved surgical technique these problems have been re-addressed and complications reduced to an acceptable range. The renewed enthusiasm for this procedure is understandable since it avoids the use of extra-genital skin grafts altogether and utilizes only urothelium, with which the urologist is certainly familiar.

Surgical technique

The bladder is catheterized and distended with fluid. Through a Pfannanstiel incision the anterior wall of the bladder is identified (Fig. 18.7) and marking sutures are placed to aid in retraction. The detrusor is incised with a scalpel or electrocautery until the mucosa is visible bulging through the incised muscle.

The graft is then obtained either by dissecting the muscle off the underlying mucosa without entering the bladder or by entering the bladder and then dissecting the graft from one side of the incision. The length of the graft should be approximately 1.5 times the urethral defect to be replaced to allow for shrinkage while handling (Fig. 18.8). After removing the graft the bladder is closed over a suprapubic catheter to provide urinary diversion. No attempt need be made to cover the area denuded of mucosa since it readily re-epithelializes.

The graft is then tubularized as for a skin graft, with the mucosal surface inwards, using a 6/0 or 7/0 absorbable suture in a running inverting fashion (see Fig. 18.2). The graft should be kept wet with saline during its tubularization; delicate smooth forceps are recommended for handling it to avoid puncturing the mucosa. The graft is then laid in the prepared recipient bed with the suture line against the corpora and anastomosed in the same manner as with a skin graft.

While there has yet to be a study on the healing process of bladder mucosal grafts, it seems likely that the stages of healing must be similar to those of free skin grafts.

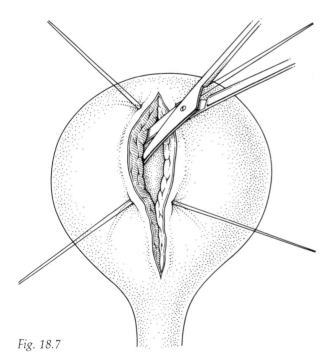

Fig. 18.7

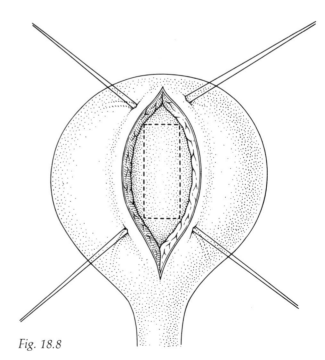

Fig. 18.8

CONCLUSION

Re-operative urethral reconstruction is a technically demanding procedure requiring a thorough knowledge of tissue healing as well as precise and delicate surgical technique. Free graft from distant extra-genital sites, to create a neo-urethra, is a concept which has stood the test of time and is certainly a viable option in some of these difficult situations. The techniques utilized in a free graft urethroplasty should be familiar to any surgeon contemplating re-operative urethral reconstruction.

REFERENCES

Converse J M, Brauer R O 1964 Transplantation of skin. In: Converse J M (ed) Reconstructive and plastic surgery, vol 1. W B Saunders, Philadelphia, chap 2, p 21

Corps B V M 1969 The effect of graft thickness, donor site and graft bed on graft shrinkage in the hooded rat. British Journal of Plastic Surgery 22: 125

Devine C J, Horton C E 1961 A one stage hypospadias repair. Journal of Urology 85: 166

Humby G 1941 A one stage operation for hypospadias. British Journal of Surgery 29: 84

McCormack R M 1954 Simultaneous chordee repair and urethral reconstruction for hypospadias. Plastic and Reconstructive Surgery 13: 257

McIndoe A H 1937 The treatment of hypospadias. American Journal of Surgery 38(1): 176

Marshall V F 1955 Construction of urethra in hypospadias using vesical mucosal grafts. Journal of Urology 73: 335

Marshall V F, Spellman R M 1957 Construction of urethra in hypospadias using vesical mucosal grafts. Plastic and Reconstructive Surgery 20: 423

Memmelaar J 1947 Use of bladder mucosa in one stage hypospadias repair. Journal of Urology 58: 68

Nove-Josserand G 1897 Traitement de l'hypospadias, nouvelle méthode. Lyon Médécine 85: 198

Nove-Josserand G 1914 Résultats éloignés de l'ureteroplastie. Journal d'Urologie 5: 393

Young F, Benjamin J 1949 Preschool age repair of hypospadias with free inlay skin graft. Surgery 26(3): 384

Chapter 19

Megalourethra

J. H. Johnston

Introduction

Congenital megalourethra is seen in two forms: the fusiform and the scaphoid (Stephens 1963).

In the fusiform type there is a severe deficiency, or even total absence, of erectile tissue in the corpora cavernosa and the corpus spongiosum. The penis is flabby, with redundant wrinkled skin, and is excessively long. Other genitourinary and ano-rectal anomalies commonly co-exist, as may the prune belly syndrome. No treatment to the megalourethra is appropriate during childhood. In survivors to adult life, the insertion of a penile prosthesis may be possible to allow sexual activity.

With scaphoid megalourethra the corpora cavernosa are normal, but there is a lack of spongy tissue in the corpus spongiosum of varied severity which leads to various degrees of dilatation of the penile urethra. The penis shows a dorsal curvature with ventral swelling, which is particularly evident during micturition. In addition, the penis is longer than average. On occasion there is a congenital fistula in the thin urethral floor. The condition is commonly a manifestation of the prune belly syndrome; even when the abdominal wall is normal and the testes are descended, the characteristic dysmorphic anomalies of the urinary tract are frequently present, so urological investigation is indicated routinely.

Treatment of the scaphoid megalourethra is needed mainly for cosmetic reasons and then only in more severe degrees of the anomaly.

SURGICAL TECHNIQUE

A circumferential skin incision is made around the penis just proximal to the corona glandis (Fig. 19.1).

The skin is dissected from the penis and the dilated urethra to the penile base (Fig. 19.2).

The floor of the megalourethra is incised longitudinally. Redundant urethral tissue is excised from each side (Fig. 19.3), leaving a strip of appropriate width between the proximal and distal urethral orifices.

The urethral strip is tubularized using interrupted fine catgut or Dexon sutures (Fig. 19.4).

The retracted skin is drawn forwards and sutured to the pericoronal fringe (Fig. 19.5).

With the above technique the urethral and cutaneous suture lines do not overlap so that there is no risk of a postoperative urethro-cutaneous fistula.

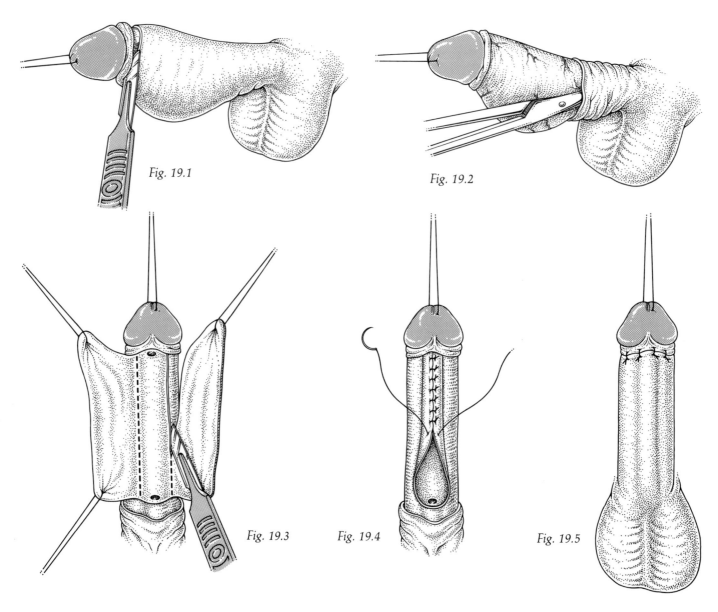

Fig. 19.1

Fig. 19.2

Fig. 19.3

Fig. 19.4

Fig. 19.5

REFERENCES

Stephens F D 1963 Congenital malformations of the rectum, anus and genito-urinary tract. Churchill Livingstone, London

Chapter 20

Circumcision

J. H. Johnston

Introduction

Phimosis is defined as the condition in which the prepuce cannot be retracted completely behind the glans penis. In the young infant this is a normal state of affairs because of congenital adhesions between the foreskin and the glans. The adhesions ordinarily separate spontaneously or with a little digital assistance during the third to fourth years of life and the prepuce then becomes readily retractable. While the child is in nappies the prepuce protects the glans against ammoniacal excoriation, so infantile circumcision has no indications on medical grounds.

The main indication for circumcision during childhood is in the boy, usually aged 6–12 years, who reports with symptoms of difficult and painful micturition with ballooning of the prepuce and in whom the preputial orifice is found to be severely fibrotic and stenotic. The pathogenesis of the condition is obscure; Rickwood et al (1980) found that the histological appearances in the prepuce were those of balanitis xerotica obliterans. Circumcision is indicated. Plastibell and similar devices have no application in this age group and excisional surgery is needed. The operation must not be regarded as a trivial one which can be left to the most inexperienced member of the surgical team. Its safe and cosmetically satisfactory performance requires an unhurried technique under general anaesthetic and the help of an assistant.

SURGICAL TECHNIQUE

The prepuce is drawn distally by an artery forceps applied to the orifice. While the skin on the shaft is pulled proximally, a circumferential incision is made just behind the corona glandis (Fig. 20.1).

The incision is deepened and the longitudinally running vessels are divided and ligated with 4/0 Dexon or catgut (Fig. 20.2).

An artery forceps grasps each side of the preputial opening on its dorsal aspect. After ensuring by gentle probing that the prepuce is freed from the glans, the prepuce is divided longitudinally by scissors (Fig. 20.3).

A nylon traction suture is placed through the glans and the divided foreskin is retracted proximally (Fig. 20.4). A circumferential incision is made through the inner layer of the prepuce some 3 mm behind the corona.

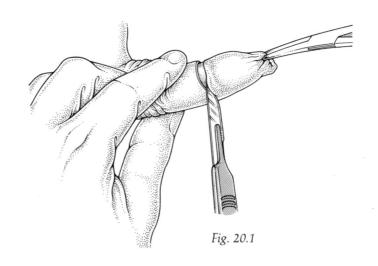

Fig. 20.1

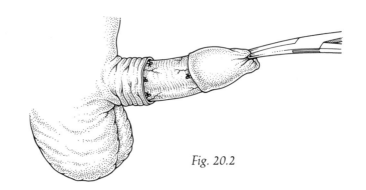

Fig. 20.2

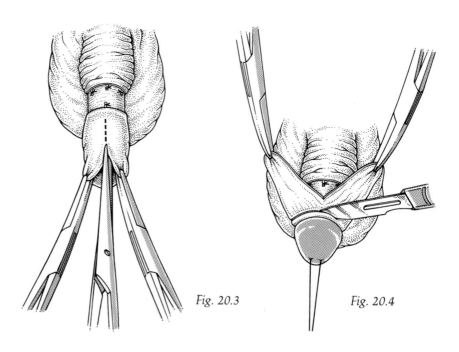

Fig. 20.3   *Fig. 20.4*

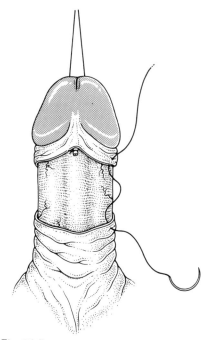

Fig. 20.5

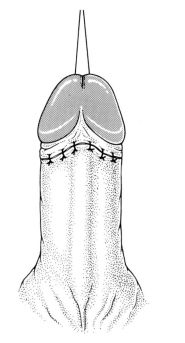

Fig. 20.6

The divided fraenal artery is ligated and the freed prepuce is excised (Fig. 20.5).

The skin edges are united with interrupted absorbable 4/0 Dexon or catgut sutures so that their later removal is not required (Fig. 20.6).

COMMENT

The use of unipolar diathermy coagulation of vessels has been regarded as dangerous during penile surgery. However, the method can be safely employed for haemostasis as an alternative to vessel ligation provided that the penile shaft is kept in contact with the body parietes whilst the current is applied. Alternatively, bipolar diathermy may be safely used.

Probably every surgeon has his own preferred dressing after penile surgery. In the present author's experience, the loose application of a 1 inch wide gauze strip soaked in Tinct. Benzoin Co. has been highly satisfactory. One week after the operation, the then hardened dressing is softened and removed while the patient is in a warm bath.

COMPLICATIONS

Complications of circumcision should be few and rare. Gross errors, such as excising too little of the inner preputial layer, causing recurrent phimosis, or removal of too much of the outer penile skin which, in extreme cases, may lead to an acquired microphallus, should be readily avoidable by the experienced surgeon.

If the prepuce is very closely adherent to the glans, even very gentle freeing may not prevent some eroding of the glandular epithelium, resulting in ulceration and later granulations. Healing occurs spontaneously within 2—3 weeks.

The surgeon should avoid tying the skin sutures (Fig. 20.6) too tightly. Otherwise an unsightly 'pie-crust' appearance can result.

REFERENCES

Rickwood A M K, Hemalatha V, Batcup G, Spitz L 1980 Phimosis in boys. British Journal of Urology 52: 147—150

Chapter 21

Urethral prolapse

J. H. Johnston

Introduction

Urethral mucosal prolapse in young girls may develop following a bout of coughing or straining at defecation, or may be encountered in an otherwise healthy child. The condition is much commoner in black children than in caucasians. The prolapsed mucosa becomes engorged and haemorrhagic so that vulval bleeding is the usual presenting symptom and a neoplasm may be simulated.

Treatment depends on the chronicity of the lesion.

SURGICAL TECHNIQUE

In the acute phase a catgut ligature can be tied around the base of the prolapse over an indwelling Foley catheter until the redundant tissue sloughs off (Fig. 21.1).

In longer-standing cases the oedematous mucosa becomes fibrotic so that its necrosis by ligature strangulation is not possible. It must be excised, preferably using diathermy as indicated in Figure 21.2.

After resection of the redundant tissue, the edges of the remaining urethral mucosa are sutured to the surrounding vulval mucosa using fine catgut or Dexon (Fig. 21.3).

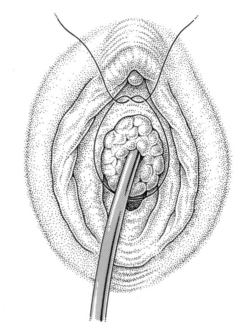

Fig. 21.1

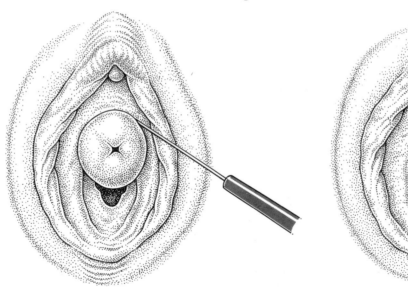

Fig. 21.2   *Fig. 21.3*

Chapter 22

Concealed (buried) penis

J. H. Johnston

Introduction

In obese boys a normal penis may appear to be abnormally short because of fat deposits over the pubis. Treatment is concerned with reduction of body weight.

True concealed penis is a congenital anomaly in which the skin is unattached to the shaft of a normally formed and sized organ so that, at first sight, the penis may even appear to be entirely absent. Figure 22.1 shows a sagittal section through genitalia to illustrate true concealed penis. Phimosis commonly co-exists. The scrotum and testes are clinically normal. Devine et al (1984) considered that the condition is due to the presence of dysgenetic fibrous bands extending from the penis to the fascia over the lower abdominal wall; however, whether the bands are the cause or the result of the deformity is arguable.

In the differential diagnosis epispadias must be considered, since on occasions the clinical appearance may be similar (Johnston 1982). With micropenis the organ is abnormally short and slender and other anomalies related to primary or secondary prenatal testicular failure co-exist. With primary insufficiency of the testes, the gonads are impalpable clinically; with secondary failure, due to disorders of the hypothalamic–pituitary axis, there are obvious gross physical defects in other systems and, in addition, severe mental retardation (Johnston 1982).

Lesser degrees of concealed penis presenting in infancy may improve spontaneously with growth, and in such cases an expectant attitude may be appropriate. With severe cases operative correction is needed and is preferably carried out before school age in order to avoid subsequent embarrassment to the patient.

SURGICAL TECHNIQUE

With the skin drawn back and a traction suture through the glans (Fig. 22.2) a circumferential incision is made around the base of the penis and deepened, with ligation and division of the subcutaneous vessels, to expose the tunicae albuginea of the corpora. The skin incision is then re-sutured, using fine nylon or Dexon and picking up the penile tunicae so that the scar becomes attached to the shaft (Figs. 22.3, 22.4 and 22.5). Figure 22.5 shows a sagittal section through genitalia after operation.

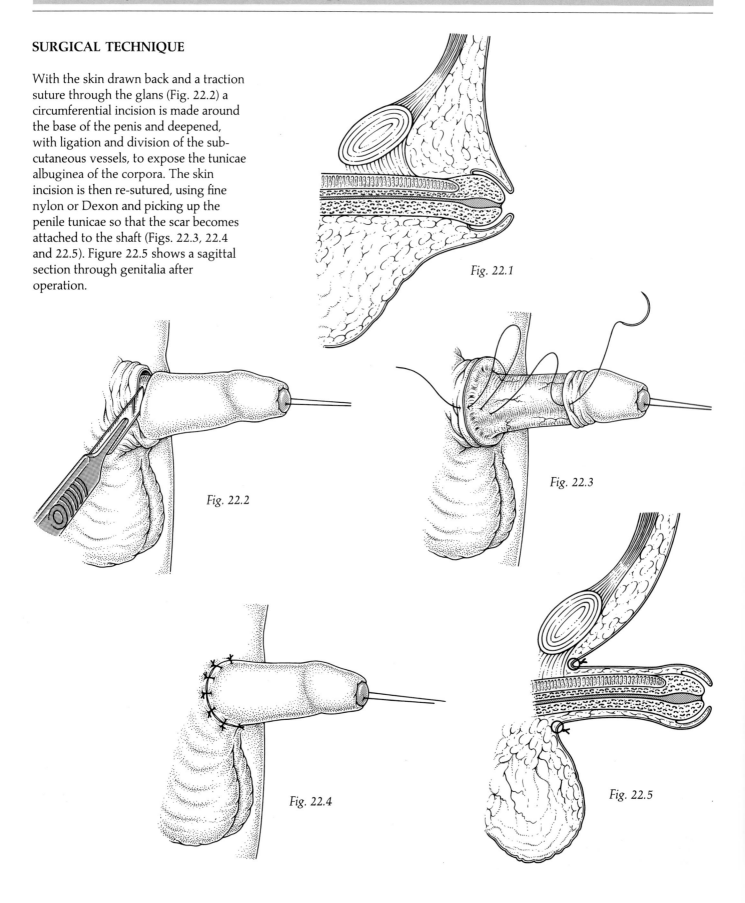

Fig. 22.1

Fig. 22.2

Fig. 22.3

Fig. 22.4

Fig. 22.5

The results of surgery are cosmetically very satisfactory although it may subsequently be found that the penile skin is somewhat redundant circumferentially; appropriate secundum artem trimming is then required after an interval of some months.

Following a circular incision around the base of the penis, the penile skin derives its blood supply from vessels originating in the coronal region. Consequently, circumcision should not be carried out at the same time as correction of the buried penis.

REFERENCES

Devine C V, Jordan G H, Horton C E 1984 Concealed penis. Society for Pediatric Urology Newsletter, November 14
Johnston J H 1982 Paediatric urology. Williams D I, Johnston J H (eds), 2nd edn. Butterworths, London, p 305, 438

Chapter 23

Webbed penis

J. H. Johnston

Introduction

The skin on the anterior surface of the scrotum extends as a sagitally disposed fold onto the ventrum of the penis. The anomaly causes no symptoms during childhood but can lead to sexual difficulties in adult life, so its correction is indicated.

SURGICAL TECHNIQUE

With traction sutures through the glans penis and the edge of the skin fold, the web is divided longitudinally to the base of the penis (Fig. 23.1).

The skin is resutured (Fig. 23.2).

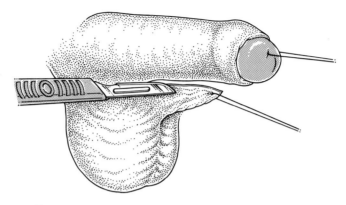

Fig. 23.1

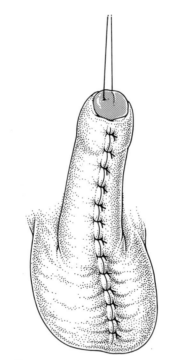

Fig. 23.2

Chapter 24

Torsion of the penis

J. H. Johnston

Introduction

Torsion of the penis around its long axis is commonly associated with lesser degrees of hypospadias. An abnormally short skin raphe lies on the right lateral aspect of the organ so that the ventrum of the penis is directed towards the patient's left side. The deformity is due solely to abnormal skin attachments and not to any defects in the penile corpora. Minor degrees of torsion require no specific treatment, but when the rotation reaches 90°, operation is indicated.

SURGICAL TECHNIQUE

A circumferential incision is made around the base of the penis to the level of the corporal tunicae (Fig. 24.1); a considerable degree of spontaneous correction is then evident.

Complete elimination of the torsion is achieved by turning the penis into proper alignment and resuturing the skin edges (Fig. 24.2). A few trial and error stitches are advisable before the suture line is finalized.

As with operation for the buried penis, surgery to the penile extremity, such as for hypospadias repair, should be deferred for several months following correction of torsion in order to ensure preservation of skin vascularity.

An alternative technique is to make the encircling skin incision around the distal penis just proximal to the urethral meatus. The skin is then freed proximally to the penile base, the torsion corrected and the incision resutured. The disadvantage of this method is that the resulting scar may interfere with the later repair of the hypospadias.

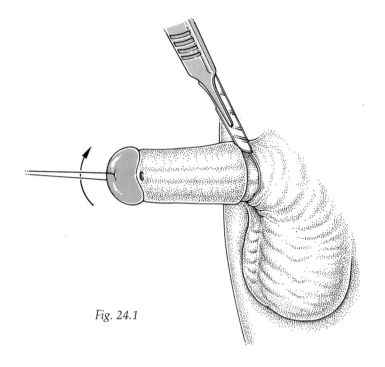

Fig. 24.1

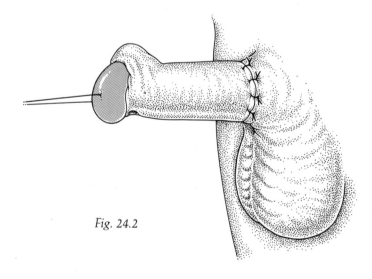

Fig. 24.2